LOSE WEIGHT

with the

CALIFORNIA CALCIUM COUNTDOWN

Unlocking Hidden Powers to Help You:

—Shed unwanted pounds—quickly and naturally

—Maintain a slim, healthy weight always

—Squash food cravings before they start

—Free yourself from addictions to food, caffeine, and nicotine

Betty Kamen, PhD

Nutrition Encounter, Novato, CA

www.bettykamen.com

All of the facts in this book have been very care-
fully researched and have been drawn from the
scientific literature. In no way, however, are any of
the suggestions meant to take the place of advice
given by physicians. Please consult a medical or
health professional should the need for one be
indicated.

Nutrition Encounter
PO Box 5847
Novato, CA 94948-5847
(415) 883-5154

Website: www.bettykamen.com
Email: betty@well.com

2004

Printed in the United States of America
First Printing 2004

ISBN 0-944501-18-4

DEDICATED

to

Perle Kinney

who understands

the full meaning of friendship

~~~~~

ACKNOWLEDGMENTS

Special thanks to these wonderful people

for their caring and sharing:

Sam Case
David Hennessy
Sam Barry
Paul Kamen
Si Kamen
Stephen A Levine, PhD

Cover Design
Raylene Buehler

ABOUT BETTY KAMEN

Years ago, on her popular radio program in New York City, Betty Kamen alerted her listeners to dozens of newly available supplements and treatments. Her program quickly developed into a center for disseminating innovative research and discoveries, featuring interviews with prominent alternative health care pioneers from around the world. Betty has written many cutting-edge health books, including the bestselling *Hormone Replacement Therapy, Yes or No? How to Make an Informed Decision* and *New Facts About Fiber.*

She received her MA in psychology in 1949, an MA in nutrition education in 1979, and her PhD in nutrition education in 1982. Betty taught at Hofstra University, developed a nutrition workshop at Stanford University Continuing Education Program for Doctors and Nurses, and served as nutrition consultant on the Committee of the Accrediting Council for Continuing Education and Training, Washington, DC.

A columnist for many health publications over the years, Betty has had hundreds of nutrition reports published. Articles written by or about Betty have appeared in the *New York Times, Chicago Tribune, San Francisco Progress, Prevention Magazine, Baltimore Sun,* and many other local and national publications. A full page photo of Betty and one of her grandchildren appeared in the March 1998 issue of *Time Magazine.*

But never mind all the credentials. Betty says her children describe her most aptly when they say, "Mom? She's just the oldest health nut in the country" — to which Betty responds: "If you have to be the oldest anything, 'health nut' is not so bad."

ONE-LINE ONLINE DAILY NUTRITION HINTS

Free!

Betty's free Table Talk nutrition hint-of-the-day has been an overwhelming success. She e-mails a free online, brief, one-line daily Table Talk Nutrition Hint if you e-mail a request to betty@well.com. Just write "hint" in the subject area. It's free!

The last ten hints, with expanded information and source references, are always available at the website:
www.bettykamen.com

Betty navigates the current medical journal reports from the world over to bring you the very latest nutrition information. You can use the daily hints as a general learning tool, or to show to your physician should any apply to your particular health challenge, if you have one. Even traditional practitioners tend to be much more open to new ideas when they are supported by a peer-reviewed study in a respected medical journal.

Ultimately, however, we must all be our own doctors (or at the very least, our own dieticians and exercise coaches), and we must make our own choices. The daily hints help us to do that.

In his beautful book, *The Fragile Species*, Lewis Thomas said, "The transformation of a society's nutrition has a greater potential for the improvement of human health than any other aspect of modern technology."

Also From Betty Kamen

~ **Betty Kamen's 1,001 Health Secrets**
What the latest research reveals about
living longer, living healthier, living better

~ **Everything I Know About Nutrition I Learned from Barley**
A guide to nutraceuticals and functional foods

~ **She's Gotta Have It**
The essential sex health manual every woman
must read

~ **The Remarkable Healing Power of Velvet Antler**
Nature's link to arthritis relief, vitality, growth
factors, sexual function, immune enhancement,
athletic performance

~ **Hormone Replacement Therapy: Yes or No?**
How to make an informed decision about
estrogen, progesterone and other strategies
for dealing with PMS, menopause and
osteoporosis

~ **Kamut: An Ancient Food for a Healthy Future**
A grain leading the green revolution for easy
access to vitamins, minerals, enzymes and
hormone precursors

~ **Everything You Always Wanted to Know About Potassium But Were Too Tired to Ask**
How potassium affects fatigue, high blood
pressure, the aging process, alcoholism, headaches
and more

Contents

Chapter One

THE SKINNY ON FAT

OBSTRUCTIONS TO WEIGHT LOSS

Wouldn't you know it – the only place you can be sure of losing weight as a natural result of the aging process is in your brain. (You lose about three ounces over the years.[1] No place else, sorry!) When it comes to the rest of your body, weight loss is up to you. Or is it?

We all know that trying to fit exercise and good nutrition into everyday life is a struggle. That's why I found the concepts that propelled me to write this book intriguing. Although there is no magic bullet, with the *California Calcium Countdown* I discovered that I could lose weight without changing my lifestyle. The amazing quick and safe fix that curtailed my food cravings also worked for my allergic sneezing spells – much to my surprise and delight!

The deeper I studied, the clearer it became that the influences working against weight control are more extensive than I had ever imagined, and they affect us through an overwhelming number of pathways. Insulin sensitivity (explained later) is one significant factor.[2] Nutrient absorption is another. Hormonal balance is yet another. Men with high uric acid levels are more likely to experience weight gain in later years.[3] Abdominal fat increases with age, a natural course of events.[4] Those with hypertension appear to be at greater risk of rebound weight gain (regaining weight lost, referred to as "yo-yo dieting").[5]

Obesity may be characterized by a low-grade inflammation because a particular substance (C-reactive protein) is elevated in those who are overweight.[6] Women are more inclined to become overweight because they give in to carbohydrate craving, whereas for men it may be bread, sausage, or other meat.[7] Brain circuits involved in cravings and addictions are normal circuits that become activated to a greater degree.[8] Even something as simple as the time of day of food intake influences overall consumption and therefore your weight![9] Sadly, the list of weight-loss hindrances appears to continue ad infinitum.

Some people are so weight-sensitive that they experience negative physical consequences with even small weight gains, while others can realize very positive effects from small weight losses.[10] These issues are very complex and go far beyond the frustrations of having a gloomy self-image because you are overweight.

There is no such thing as being perfectly healthy and *somewhat* overweight – that's like being just a *little bit* pregnant. Most of us know that overweight people are subject to two-to-four times the risk of heart disease, high blood pressure, stroke, cancer, and diabetes.[11] Less obvious is that overweight people also have:

> ~ heightened sensitivity to pain
> ~ increased health risk during surgery
> ~ more abdominal hernias
> ~ enhanced risk for degenerative arthritis
> ~ greater incidence of cholesterol gallstones
> ~ lipid (blood fat) abnormalities
> ~ accelerated mortality after middle age
> ~ sleep-disordered breathing
> ~ higher recurrence rates of prostate cancer
> after radical prostatectomy
> ~ increased potential for depression
> ~ pregnancy complications[12,13,14,15,16,17,18]

Not as serious, but occurring even in those who are overweight by as little as ten pounds, the list of symptoms continues with more dandruff, hemorrhoids, flat feet, varicose veins, psychological complaints, dental decay, and slower growth of nails and hair.[19]

With the promise of better health in so many areas and even longer life at the end of the dieting rainbow as motivation, you would think we would all be highly fired up to stick to a diet. But it turns out that powerful forces are at work – forces no different from those at work for people who smoke, don't buckle their seatbelt, are compulsive shoppers, gamblers or talkers, use dangerous recreational drugs, or even risk life-threatening sexually transmitted diseases.

A yearlong study was conducted in which physicians trained patients to promote an approach to obesity treatment through lifestyle modification. When the project was completed, the researchers concluded that the twelve-month program was a complete failure. *None of the participants lost weight after all that extensive personal attention and professional coaching.*[20]

Genetics are no help, either. They have played only a secondary role in the rising prevalence of obesity. Scientists agree that the most important determinants of the increasing adiposity worldwide appear to have been the environmental factors affecting diet and activity. This is never more obvious than when we take a walk through a mall and compare the ratio of those who are acceptably thin to those who are overweight.

Many who are overweight resist medical care because they are not happy about exposing their bodies to the doctors and nurses. They know the gowns are too small, they can't squeeze into waiting room chairs, exam tables tip over, and some procedures require extra staff to lift their middle.[21]

Meanwhile, hospitals are buying expensive new equipment such as reinforced toilets, oversized beds, larger blood pressure cuffs, wider and better reinforced wheelchairs, and bigger versions of other basic supplies to treat the growing number of people who are overweight by at least 100 pounds. Longer surgical gloves, needles and syringes are now standard. One funeral company even has a line of expanded caskets to meet the need.[22]

A physician was advised to take his patient to the National Zoo for her MRI because she would not fit into the hospital's equipment.

Another doctor was forced to take a patient to a loading dock for a weight appraisal. Yet another patient was lifted onto a stretcher by the fire department's hoisting equipment.

My closest friend weighs in at 290 pounds (at least that's all she'll admit to). When she gets the observation from a caregiver, **"My, you *are* overweight…"**, she responds, **"I'd like a second opinion."** After the caregiver's embarrassed laughter, the dialogue becomes more meaningful.

OTHER FATTENING FACTORS

Following are additional stumbling blocks that impede our efforts to lose those extra pounds:

~ Fat cells are very economical and efficient in energy storage. We have inherited the ability to stockpile fat easily, providing energy to hunt for food and to face those saber-toothed tigers – an attribute necessary for life itself throughout most of human existence. Like some treasure placed in a vault, this "message" has never left our DNA – perhaps not through millions of years of time.

~ That same ancestry includes a design for survival in a different environment – effective for an era when it was common to miss food for long periods, an era that was pre-agricultural, pre-farming, pre-supermarket, pre-three-meals-a-day. We are simply not genetically programmed for an overabundance of easily available donuts.

~ We are a pleasure-seeking society. It's hard for most of us to give up an immediate indulgence for a future benefit. We are programmed to respond to instant gratification without consideration of distant potential problems.

~ Humans prefer sweets long before birth. Even a five-month-old human fetus increases its swallowing rate when a sweetener is injected into the amniotic fluid of the mother.[23] (And let's not forget the popular phrase, "This baby is as sweet as sugar.")

~ The "sweet reward" is universal; it is part of every culture, and is offered as a bonus for special behavior, or as a stress-reliever, but not necessarily to satisfy hunger. In the workplace, coffee breaks and meetings replete with sugar-laden goodies have become national institutions. At this very moment, bands of very highly-paid chemists around the world are competing with each other to find the best natural substance to make life even "sweeter" for you.

~ The distance between a natural (or "real") food and the food we encounter on our table has widened, and continues to do so. The calories consumed with foods that have not been tampered with are self-limiting. Not so with processed foods.

~ We frequently eat comfort foods in an attempt to reduce chronic stress responses.[24] (It's been said that if all fast food restaurants disappeared overnight, the scales would still point to obesity because we would find food elsewhere to satisfy emotional needs.)

~ Feedback systems signal our brains to seek food when our body *thinks* it is needed, not necessarily when it is actually needed.

~ Our likes and dislikes affect our metabolism. An unpleasant taste stimulus (like broccoli for President Bush, Sr.) has a significantly different effect on the kind and volume of pancreatic flow than a pleasant stimulus (like broccoli for me).[25]

~ We tend to binge, uncurbed, when a behavior-regulating neurotransmitter called *serotonin* is out of order. (Neurotransmitters are vehicles for communication between our nerve cells.) The result is excessive consumption of refined carbohydrates and/or cravings for sweets.[26,27]

~ Weight gain may be a side effect of prescription medication. In almost no instance does the weight come off easily when the drug is discontinued.[28]

~ Weight gain may also be a side effect of certain disease states. These include hypothyroidism, Cushing's syndrome, growth hormone and testosterone deficiency, polycystic ovarian syndrome, and hypothalamic lesions.[29]

~ From fast food outlets in the US, Mexico and Brazil to restaurants in Singapore and grocery stores in Britain, the size of food portions, chocolate bars and beverages has expanded (along with the size of those who consume them). Walloping portions encourage people to eat more. And big portions of *calorie-dense food* – the kind people tend to grab on the run – boost calorie consumption even higher without providing additional satisfaction. Big portions of high-calorie foods put people at greater risk of overeating than big portions of unprocessed foods.[30]

PORTLY PORTIONS

A bagel 20 years ago was 3 inches in diameter and had 140 calories. Today's 6-inch bagel has 350 calories. A 6.9-ounce portion of french fries has 610 calories, 400 more than the typical 2.4-ounce portion 20 years ago.

~ Many people who have allergies have difficulty controlling their weight. The problem is one of biochemical internal disarray, which interferes with our natural "set point," the point at which our body wants to maintain its weight. Our complex brain tries unsuccessfully to sort this out, along with other confusing messages. (This metabolic mishap will be discussed in detail, and is a very significant factor involved in fad-diet failures.)

Is it any wonder that it's so difficult to lose weight? With so many factors working against us, what can we do? I believe that the *California Calcium Countdown* can work *with* many of these factors, not *against* them, including our pesky Paleolithic fat-protective legacy.

MORE FAT FACTS

~ The number of people who are clinically obese has soared to more than 300 million globally, and one billion are overweight, with an estimated 2.5 million dying every year. The World Health Organization now lists obesity among the top ten health concerns in the world. The related health risks are putting enormous stress on national healthcare systems worldwide.[31]

~ At any given time, 29 percent of men and 44 percent of women in the US are trying to lose weight. That means nearly 45 million Americans are actively dieting every year.[32] In the European Union, overweight and obese people account for over 50,000 "avoidable" cases of cancer annually, 9,000 of which are in the United Kingdom alone.[33]

~ Obesity can be divided into two classifications – *hyperplastic*, which refers to increased *numbers* of fat cells, and *hypertrophic*, which pertains to increased *size* of fat cells (the same number of cells, just fatter ones).

~ The medical definition of obesity is based on the amount of body fat a person has. A person can weigh more than what is thought to be healthy without being obese. For example: A person may weigh too much because his or her body retains too much water, a condition referred to as edema, which, nevertheless causes that person to look obese. Some athletes may weigh more than what is normally considered a healthy weight because their excess weight is muscle, not fat.

~ People are not always overweight because of lack of exercise. Of course exercise is a factor, and yes, exercise is beneficial; it helps us to absorb nutrients more efficiently. But exercise is not the *only* factor.

~ The more pounds that overweight men trying to lose weight shed, the more likely they are to keep those pounds off. Men who lose the most weight are less likely to regain it than are those who lose only moderate amounts.[34]

~ Hypertension in the US increased during the 1990s and now affects more than a quarter of the adult population. More than half the increase is due to an increase in weight.[35]

~ Fat is distributed differently in men and women. Coronary calcification increases more in women with diabetes than in men because of this difference.[36]

~ Disability has increased, not among the elderly, but among those under 50. Obesity accounts for about half the increased disability among those aged 18 to 29.[37]

~ Despite enormous effort, the pharmaceutical industry has not yet come up with an acceptable weight-loss drug solution mainly because most weight-loss drugs have serious adverse effects on health and well-being.[38]

~ Those who experience greater weight loss also experience correspondingly greater improvements in health-related quality of life.[39]

~ The FDA has been brainstorming for ideas to combat the trend toward obesity that it blames for 300,000 deaths a year and $117 billion in increased medical costs and lost productivity. So far, none of their ideas has worked.

~~~~~

Julie Gerberding, Director of the Centers for Disease Control and Prevention, Atlanta, said, "Americans are much more likely to die from cancer, heart disease, and diabetes caused by smoking, **eating too much** and exercising too little, rather than anthrax, smallpox, or diseases like SARS (Severe Acute Respiratory Syndrome) and West Nile virus infection."[40] In other words fat can be, and often is, fatal.

Since the major causes of death and disease are preventable, the information in *California Calcium Countdown* should raise your hopes and your health.

MEMOS

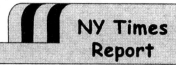

NY Times Report

The New York Times,
January 20, 2004

When shopping for clothes, you may notice that your clothing size keeps dropping even though you know you've put on a few pounds. Size inflation is the term being used this year to explain the change in clothing sizes. Basically, the clothes keep getting bigger, but the numbers stay the same. For example, today's size four is actually a size eight. Retailers know that people are gaining weight; they also know consumers want to wear as small a size as possible, so they're meeting that desire.

Similarly in the restaurant industry, after a complaint from an oversized customer, the president of a popular restaurant chain ordered bigger chairs to accommodate oversized customers so they wouldn't dine elsewhere.

Chapter Two

CAUSES OF
CALCIUM MALABSORPTION

BACKGROUND

In 1984, The Haight-Ashbury Free Medical Clinic in San Francisco was searching for something that would help treat patients who were seriously addicted to stimulant drugs and alcohol. In response to the request, Stephen A. Levine, PhD, a biochemist and founder of Allergy Research Group, developed a special product. (Allergy Research Group is a supplement manufacturing company in Hayward, California, meeting the needs of physicians.) Dr. Levine's compound curtailed these cravings almost dead in their tracks! The longer the participants used the formula – which was natural and free of side effects – the more benefit they derived.

The product worked fast – in fact, within minutes. Nor was a large quantity necessary for the positive results. The average intake was only 1½ teaspoons per day. (See Appendix A for excerpts of this successful study, titled "Efficacy of Buffered Ascorbate Compound (BAC) in the Detoxification and Aftercare of Clients Involved in Opiate and Stimulant Abuse.")

The scientists taking part in the project conjectured that if this formula could achieve such striking and powerful effects on critically addicted people, surely it could help those struggling against powerful food cravings. After all, they reasoned, the metabolic pathways involved in the addiction or cravings for fat and sugar are comparable to those of most addictive drugs.[1]

Experts in the field note that it's more than a linguistic accident that the same term – *craving* – is used to describe intense desires for both foods and for a variety of drugs of abuse.[2]

With mounting evidence to support the parallel mechanisms between drug/alcohol abuse and excessive craving for sweets and fattening foods, the product was made available to physicians and caregivers for general patient use. Glowing reports have been accumulating ever since. I have used the product for years, mainly to keep two allergic symptoms under control, but it never occurred to me that it could have been credited for keeping my weight close to where I wanted it.

I now understand that this nutrient-dense, non-drug product helps to create a sense of satiety – a feeling of being full, the kind of feeling that says, "I'm really not hungry. I don't need that slice of cheesecake."

Sound too good to be true? **Read on.**

The original product was comprised of buffered vitamin C along with the minerals potassium, calcium, and magnesium. The current version includes vitamin C extracted from a unique cassava root source, which makes the mix easily tolerated by those who have difficulty with extracts of vitamin C from other derivations. And, like the old formula, the new blend contains the same minerals, but it has been enhanced with vitamin D3, vitamin K and a few proprietary additions.

How these nutrients work synergistically to elicit a lean-body advantage is explained later. Stirred into liquid, the combination makes a sparkling, effervescent drink. The carbonates of potassium, calcium and magnesium give the product an acid/alkaline buffering action (pH 7.0 in water – also explained later), potentially improving bowel tolerance and minimizing hyperacidity.

THE EXPERTS WEIGH IN:
VALIDATION FROM MEDICAL JOURNALS

Currently, the weight-loss effect of calcium – one of the key ingredients in this formula – has been receiving a great deal of attention. More exciting is the fact that reliable scientific research has been catching up with the observations. It has become perfectly clear that calcium expedites weight loss, even in the presence of high-fat diets. Note the following:

~ From the *Journal of Nutrition*:
Growing evidence supports a relationship between increased calcium intakes and reductions in body weight.[3]

~ From the *International Journal of Obesity & Related Metabolic Disorders* and the *Journal of Biomedical Central Cardiovascular Disorders*:
A diet consisting mainly of high calcium foods resulted in an average weight loss of 24.6 pounds in 16 weeks. This is greater than the average weight loss in one year in trials using weight-loss drugs such as dexfenfluramine, sibutramine or orlistat. (Even if the drugs rivaled the calcium diet for weight loss, they have serious side effects: sibutramine increases blood pressure and pulse rate; orlistat causes gastrointestinal side effects; and dexfenfluramine results in serious heart valve diseases.)[4,5]

~ From *Lipids*:
Test animals were placed on a diet high in sucrose and increased fat, including lard. As anticipated, these animals quickly became obese. But when some of them were given high levels of calcium, they stopped gaining weight and, instead, began to lose weight. Even though the caloric intake of the two sets of animals was identical, those on a low calcium diet gained weight, while those on a high calcium diet lost weight. There are several reasons why dietary calcium can lessen weight gain

even if you are consuming a fattening meal. Among them: Calcium helps to suppress a substance that would normally increase adiposity (fat) with a calorie-dense meal. By increasing dietary calcium, the result is a significant *reduction* in adipose tissue – *without dieting* – markedly accelerating weight- and body-fat loss.[6]

~ From *Experimental Biology*:
High-calcium, low-calorie diets helped test animals lose weight at rates **double** those given low levels of calcium.[7]

~ From the *Official Publication of the Federation of American Societies for Experimental Biology (FASEB)*:
Overweight patients with high blood pressure were asked to consume two cups of yogurt daily. No other changes were made in their diet or exercise routines. An average of 10.56 pounds was lost in one year simply by adding the yogurt.[8]

~ From the *Journal of the American College of Nutrition*
Laboratory, clinical and population data all indicate a significant anti-obesity effect of dietary calcium.[9]

~ From *Obesity Research*
Research shows a higher excretion of dietary fat in the presence of high calcium.[10]

~ From the *Journal of the American College of Nutrition*:
A two-year study found that young women who had the highest intakes of calcium lost the most weight and body fat on weight-control programs, regardless of exercise level.[11]

Additional sophisticated peer-reviewed trials continue to confirm that high-calcium diets are associated with lower body weight.[12] And, in a study published in the *Journal of Nutrition*, researchers estimated that only 1,000 milligrams of additional calcium intake daily can result in a 17.6-pound difference in your body weight.[13]

Other research studies are cited on pages 40-41.

CALCIUM'S UNEXPECTED BONUS

Because of the strong association and seemingly infinite number of studies showing the relationship of calcium to bones, it took medical researchers by surprise to learn that this mineral is also a critical key to the regulation of metabolism and fat burning.

In summary, my interest in calcium and weight loss was piqued by:

~ the experience of accomplished clinical physicians who have been observing thousands of patients using this product over two decades

~ the scientific investigations that validate the calcium/weight-loss phenomenon

~ my personal success with the use of this product

With all this evidence, you can understand my enthusiasm.

Chapter seven discusses the importance of the *right* kind of calcium and its associated nutrient cofactors.

BUT WAIT A MINUTE . . .

In nature's wisdom, nutrients that our bodies require in greater quantity appear in our foods in higher amounts. Milk and milk products (and their progeny of nonfat milk solids and whey and ice cream and cheese), wheat and other grains (and their offshoot of flour used in baked goods), soy, almonds and Brazil nuts, oysters, many varieties of fish (especially sardines), egg yolk, chocolate, cocoa, molasses, broccoli, tofu, leafy greens and kidney beans contain significant quantities of calcium. Calcium abounds!

Why, then, should we require more? Why is calcium now being added to all manner of foods and drugs – from laxatives to flour to McDonald's hamburger buns to diet colas, and, in England, even to milk itself? And why aren't we all thin with all this calcium around?

HOW MUCH IS IN THERE?
Calcium In Milligrams In 100 Grams Of Food

Broccoli................100	Mustard greens...183
Cheese...................100-900	Oranges................. 41
Collards.................250	Oysters................. 90
Dried apricots...... 67	Raisins................. 62
Dried beans...........144	Salmon..................154
Dried prunes......... 90	Shrimp..................115
Eggs...................... 54	Turnip greens.......246
Kale......................240	Wheat bread........ 99
Milk......................118	

Yogurt - 8 oz cup.....314

Although other foods are lower in calcium than those listed above, they are by no means negligible. Fresh fruits, for example, are rich in calcium, but their high water content results in low percentages on a per weight basis.[14]

In a typical diet, milk, cheese, and yogurt contribute about 42 percent of total calcium intake. An additional 21 percent comes from dairy ingredients in mixed foods such as macaroni and cheese, pizza, sandwiches, and desserts. The remaining dietary calcium sources are from single grains (16 percent); vegetables (7 percent), poultry and fish (5 percent); fruit (3 percent); and miscellaneous foods (7 percent).[15]

CALCIUM: HOW MUCH IS NEEDED?

RDI is a new term that replaces the familiar Recommended Daily Allowances (RDAs). RDIs are based on a population average of the latest RDAs for vitamins and minerals for healthy Americans over 4 years of age. They are average values for the *entire* population.

Women get an average of less than 75 percent of the RDI for calcium for most of their lives, and those over fifty get less than half the RDI. Men fare slightly better, but are still 40 percent off the RDI after age fifty.

To claim any food as an excellent source of calcium, 200 milligrams or 20 percent of the US Daily Value (1,000 milligrams) of calcium is required to be in that food.[16]

According to the RDA, women older than 50 require about 1,500 milligrams per day since less calcium is absorbed as one ages.

Despite all the calcium in our diet, it only *appears* that we are consuming enough of this vital mineral. Look at the list of calcium foods on page 28, keeping in mind that processed foods are sadly depleted of their calcium content. How many of the foods listed have you ingested in an *unprocessed* form? And perhaps even more significant, what about **calcium-absorption antagonists**?

Research confirms that the majority of people do not absorb calcium efficiently. Variation in absorption explains more of the differences in calcium balance than actual calcium intake.[17]

CALCIUM CRUSHERS:
WHAT ARE CALCIUM ABSORPTION ANTAGONISTS?

Calcium is excreted in sweat and urine. In addition, the presence in the diet of the following food substances interferes with the absorption of calcium from your intestines:

~ phosphoric acid, found in protein foods, especially red meats, milk, nuts, eggs, cheese, and soft drinks
~ oxalic acid, found in raw spinach, chocolate, cocoa, coffee, most berries (especially strawberries and cranberries), most nuts (especially peanuts), and rhubarb
~ citric acid, found naturally in citrus fruits but also used as flavoring agents in many food products
~ phytic acid, found in grains, legumes, and oilseeds, and especially high in soy protein isolates

Soy has one of the highest phytate levels of any legume and, unlike others, its phytic acid is not destroyed with extended cooking time.

A few decades ago, our Food and Nutrition Board estimated that we probably absorb only about 40 percent of the calcium we ingest. That percentage would be considered high in today's world of increased processed foods and soda pop.

Another major factor influencing calcium absorption has to do with foods ingested in the same meal.

Foods that enhance the absorption of calcium are:
>   fatty fish
>   fat in foods generally, eg, eggs, butter, and liver

Foods that diminish the absorption of calcium are:
>   sodas (because of their phosphorus content)
>   unleavened bread
>   milk

Therefore, two people with the same calcium intake will absorb different amounts of calcium if one is enjoying:
>   scrambled eggs for breakfast
>   salmon salad for lunch
>   liver and onions for dinner

while the other has:
>   cornflakes and milk for breakfast
>   a diet Coke midmorning
>   a hamburger and a Pepsi for lunch
>   a soft drink with a dinner
>   a dinner of beef stew in the evening
>   pita pouches or unleavened bread daily

Both diets offer calcium of about equal quantity, but the amount of calcium that can be utilized will be very different.

Further evidence of the complexity of calcium absorption is demonstrated by the fact that despite the vast difference of calcium between cow's milk and mother's milk – cow's milk contains four times more calcium than human milk – the infant who is breastfed absorbs more calcium. The experts are still trying to sort out the mechanisms at work here.[18]

Substances concentrated in the outer layers of grain seed (such as wheat bran) may also make calcium unavailable for absorption. These substances, known as *phytates* (listed in the antagonists above), are partially destroyed in baking and in the fermentation processes.[19] (Since sprouting also destroys phytates, consuming sprouted grain breads is in your best calcium-absorption interest. These breads are sold in health food stores.)

Reducing or eliminating the fat content of milk does no favors for your calcium absorption, either. As stated, the absorption of calcium and fat are interrelated. **Small amounts of fat** *improve* **calcium absorption.**

Whole milk contains only about 3 percent fat, but reducing this amount interferes with proper calcium absorption. **Excessive amounts of fat, however, *reduce* calcium absorption.**

So drinking whole milk is better than drinking skimmed milk, but having french fries that soaked up the oils in which the potatoes are cooked is certainly not advantageous. Consuming foods in their natural form solves the problem. It is difficult to either overdose on fat or consume too little if foods are not processed.

Although you may have been led to believe that skimmed milk is a healthful diet food for diet-conscious people, it is highly processed, and as such it's a negative for calcium absorption. The alteration of its original architecture affects your calcium balance. *Butterfat is vital to adequate calcium absorption.* (As explained later, even whole milk is not in your best calcium-absorption interest.)

Here are a few additional reasons for calcium deficiencies:

~ Absorption of calcium decreases during illness.

~ Heavy reliance on processed foods limits *all* nutrient intake, including calcium.

~ If you feel stressed because your mother-in-law is intruding or because your teenager is causing you grief, your calcium is zapped. *Stress depletes calcium.*

~ Calcium absorption tends to decrease with increased age in both men and women, but the decline commences earlier for women: age forty-five for females, and sixty for men. After menopause women excrete more calcium in urine.[20]

~ Calcium absorption is impaired under conditions of vitamin D deficiency, a condition which is rampant in the US. Even individuals with vitamin D levels within the reference range but at the low end may not be getting the full benefit from their calcium intake. Researchers have concluded that the lower end of the current reference range is set too low.[21]

~ Antacids, tetracyclines, laxatives, diuretics, heparin, and other drugs impede calcium absorption.

~ Individual differences play a role. One researcher demonstrated this by studying the calcium retention of two normal five-year-olds eating the same food. One retained 78 percent more calcium than the other.

~ People who are lactose intolerant tend to get less calcium in their diets because they limit milk-based foods.[22]

~ Surgical removal of one or both ovaries, commonplace in the US, induces calcium loss.[23]

~ Chlorine (as used in almost all tap water) and fluorine in water cause calcium excretion. Sugar intake has the same effect.[24]

~ Pasteurization causes a significant loss of calcium in milk and milk products.

~ Consuming phosphorus, as found in soft drinks, has the same effect as calcium deficiency. With cola beverages, you are getting doses of phosphoric acid (also listed in our antagonists above) without any calcium. That extra phosphorus binds with calcium and prevents it from being absorbed.[25]

~ During adolescence, calcium retention is dependent on race. With the same intake, African American girls retain more calcium than Caucasian girls through increased calcium absorption, decreased excretion and increased bone formation rates.[26]

~ Aluminum, which comes from tap water, canned drinks, antacids, cooking utensils and preservatives, inhibits calcium absorption.[27]

~ Consumption of alcohol (but not wine) can contribute to calcium loss.[28]

~ There is a direct correlation between salt intake and calcium excretion.[29,30]

~ Although calcium absorption increases twofold during pregnancy, it drops to values like those for non-pregnant women when breastfeeding.[31]

Understanding how these calcium antagonists affect the body helps explain why we need supplemental calcium, and why, when our foods are awash with calcium, we are a nation marked by obesity.

Chances are you are getting a sizable amount of calcium but too much phosphorus. Foods containing phophorus are: almost all processed or canned meats (hot dogs, ham, bacon), processed cheese, baked products that use phosphate baking powder (commonly used), cola drinks and other soft drinks, instant soups and puddings, toppings and seasonings, breads, cereals, meat, potatoes, and a long list of phosphate food additives. The calcium and phosphorus flow charts on page 99 demonstrate the differences in absorption of these two minerals.

MILK IS NOT A GOOD CALCIUM SOURCE. . . BUT WHY?

Contrary to what we have been taught, milk does little to help calcium absorption. Milk and milk products are almost equal sources of both phosphorus and calcium, and sometimes contain even more phosphorus. (Cottage cheese, for example, is considerably higher in phosphorus than calcium.) At high levels of ingestion, calcium absorption decreases sharply.

Calcium is only a quick-picker-upper at low levels. Therefore, even if the same quantities of calcium and phosphorus are absorbed, the ratio shifts in favor of phosphorus.

For optimal absorption of calcium and phosphorus, both nutrients should be supplied by food in almost equal amounts, with a little more calcium than phosphorus. An abnormal calcium/phosphorus ratio interferes with the absorption of both elements and may result in calcium deficiency. The average

American diet, which is high in phosphorus, is not conducive to this one-to-one ratio. Most of our diets have a low calcium-to-phosphorus ratio, which means that we consume less calcium than phosphorus. Alfalfa, anyone? That's one of the few foods with the ideal one-to-one calcium/phosphorus ratio.

When equal amounts of phosphorus and calcium are increased, a point is reached at which resorption of calcium from your bones increases. Resorption is the process of returning some of your bone's calcium content to your blood. Your body knows that the ratio of these two minerals in your blood is critical for health, so it compensates by taking the needed calcium from the reservoir, your bones.

The reason for this is that inorganic phosphate is absorbed very efficiently at high intakes, whereas calcium is not. As indicated, at high levels of ingestion, calcium absorption decreases sharply. Therefore, even if the same quantities are absorbed, as in milk, *the ratio shifts in favor of phosphorus.*

Another problem: Although the amount of phosphorus consumed in *additive* form is highly variable, the average intake is about one-half gram every day. This additive represents an increase of 25 percent above average, and would shift your calcium-to-phosphorus ratio to one-to-three-and-a-half (1.0:3.5). In addition, phosphorus additives are inorganic, and absorption of inorganic phosphate is more efficient than the organic phosphates found naturally in foods.

As I write these pages, a member of my family came to report that the Department of Agriculture just announced that the average American consumes 38 gallons of soda a year, and that if each American consumed only 12 ounces a day, that would lower the statistics!

February 4, 2004

THE MILK MYTH: PUT THIS COW TO PASTURE

Milk loses 50 percent of its calcium during the pasteurization process. Low-fat and no-fat milk products render the calcium almost useless because, again, fat is necessary for the transportation and absorption of calcium. Americans drink more milk than the people of any other modern nation, yet we have the highest incidence of bone problems. One study found no association between consumption of milk throughout life and protection from vertebral deformities. (It was the absence of calcium later in life that made the difference.)[32]

Milk, because it is so rich in animal protein, often causes a greater calcium loss than gain – referred to as *negative calcium balance*.[33] This fact may come as a surprise, even to the professionals, who have been conditioned to believe that cow's milk is a major source of calcium.

Is it possible that America's romance with milk is due to the extensive (and biased) educational materials supplied at no cost to the public, to schools, and to professionals over the years by the dairy industry? I recently found a box of memorabilia which included a good-health certificate awarded to me in school in 1937. The certificate announced that "Betty Banoff is in good health because she drinks milk every day."

I did drink a lot of milk daily, but I was plagued with endless respiratory diseases, missing more days of school than I attended. I know now that I am lactose-intolerant, that milk for me is mucus-forming and causes inflammatory problems, and that it was a major contribution to my early ill health and teenage acne.

Because there are so many factors working against calcium absorption, fortifying widely consumed foods with calcium (as in cold cereals) has been considered. According to experts writing in the *Journal of Nutrition*, fortification of regularly selected foods is *not* a realistic way to address the issue of low calcium intakes.[34]

When calcium is not properly utilized, it deposits in various parts of your body:
> in joints, contributing to arthritis
> in arteries, promoting arteriosclerosis
> in kidneys and bladder, causing stones to form

It also calcifies, resulting in bursitis and tinnitus. (Tinnitus is characterized by sound in one or both ears, such as buzzing, ringing, or whistling, occurring without an external stimulus.)

Researchers in Northern Italy found that those who drink two or more glasses of milk a day have five times the risk of prostate cancer than those in a control group who drink no milk. Several other studies associate milk with prostate cancer.

A study that involved twenty-seven countries found a strong correlation between cow's milk and multiple sclerosis.

Infant formulas based on cow's milk have been connected to the development of type 1 diabetes in children.

A decade long study in fifteen countries concluded that drinking two glasses of milk a day increases the risk of lymphatic cancer by 3.5 time.

Theories about why these associations exist include the presence of lactose in milk, additives, and even the fact that milk has a very unbalanced ratio of calcium to magnesium of 9 to 1.

Cow's milk is a perfect food - for a calf.

In all of its physiologic actions, calcium influences and is influenced by other minerals. In our present state of ignorance about the causation of major chronic diseases, it is important for us to realize that imbalances can be the result of overzealous practices. That is why *moderate* amounts of calcium for supplementation, *only if accompanied by other nutrients*, remains the best choice. The proper balance is discussed in chapter seven.

Looking at published data describing the inverse relationship between calcium intake and body weight, respected researcher Robert Heaney concluded: "Increasing calcium intake can be estimated to reduce the prevalence of overweight . . . by perhaps as much as 60 to 80 percent."[35]

~~~~~

More than a century ago, the prevailing view was that all disease was caused by external invaders, either bacterial or toxic, so the idea that *not* eating something could make you sick was inconceivable.

Today, it may fly in the face of convention that *not* eating something (such as calcium and its cofactor nutrients in supplemental form) could also make and keep you fat!

An old philosopher once said, "Beliefs, when they are long-standing, become fixed rules of life and assume a prescriptive right not to be questioned." I hope you will consider the revolutionary plan outlined in *California Calcium Countdown*. It could have a dramatic effect on your life.

MORE STUDIES SUPPORTING CALCIUM FOR WEIGHT LOSS

~ If you are overweight and not watching your diet, increasing dietary calcium results in significant reductions in fat tissue, and if you are on a calorie-restricted diet, the calcium will accelerate your weight loss and body fat loss.

Lipids, 2003[36]

~ Growing evidence supports a relationship between increased calcium intakes and reductions in body weight specific to fat mass. The impact of calcium intake on weight loss or prevention of weight gain has been demonstrated in a wide age range of Caucasian and African-Americans of both genders.

Journal of Nutrition 2003[37]

~ Girls who consume more calcium tend to weigh less and have lower body fat than those with low calcium consumption, although it is not important whether the calcium comes from food or supplements.

Experimental Biology Meeting 2003[38]

~ Low calcium diets impede body fat loss.

Lipids 2003[39]

~ An increase in calcium consumption can reduce the risk of obesity.

International Obesity Symposium 2003[40]

Medical Hypotheses 2003[41]

Urologic Oncology 2003[42]

~ Higher levels of calcium intake may prevent fat storage, and more calcium may raise metabolism, thus burning more calories.

Southwestern Medical Center Report 2003[43]

~ Each 300 mg increment in regular calcium intake is associated with approximately 1 kg less body fat in children and 2.5–3.0 kg lower body weight in adults. Increasing calcium intake could reduce the risk of overweight substantially, perhaps by as much as 70 percent. (1 kilogram is equal to 2.2 pounds.)

Journal of the American College of Nutrition 2003[44]

~ Calcium may play a role in increasing levels of high-density lipoprotein (HDL, the good kind), reducing kidney stone recurrence, reducing symptoms of premenstrual syndrome, and promoting weight loss.

Urology in Nursing 2003[45]

~ Women at midlife gain an average of about one pound a year (with one-sixth of them gaining at the rate of 2.5 pounds a year) *if they are on low calcium intakes.* By contrast, women who take the RDI amount of calcium show a slight negative weight gain each year.

Journal of Clinical Endocrinology & Metabolism 2000 [46]

Chapter Three

EATING BEHAVIOR: CRAVINGS AND ADDICTIONS

Volumes have been written about chocolate cravings, and it is a frequent topic of conversation. My sister and I still laugh about this incident, which occurred many years ago, and typifies the message in this chapter.

Dec. 5th -- afternoon
Me:
What did Vic give you for your birthday?

My sister:
A HUGE box of chocolates.

Dec. 5th. -- evening
My sister:
I couldn't resist the chocolate. Almost all of it is gone - in one day! Oh, my poor stomach.

Me:
Put the rest in the freezer. Out of sight, out of mind.

Dec. 6th. -- morning
My sister (with sarcasm):
Thanks a lot for your suggestion. I enjoyed the frozen chocolates even more.

FAT, SUGAR, TEXTURE, & AROMA

Although addictive behavior is generally associated with drug and alcohol abuse or compulsive sexual activity, chocolate may evoke similar psychopharmacologic and behavioral reactions in susceptible persons. The hedonic appeal of chocolate (fat, sugar, texture, and aroma) is a predominant factor in such cravings.

Other characteristics of chocolate, however, may be equally important contributors to the phenomena of chocolate cravings. Chocolate may be used by some as a form of self-medication for dietary deficiencies (eg, magnesium) or to balance low levels of neurotransmitters involved in the regulation of mood, food intake, and compulsive behaviors.

Chocolate cravings are often episodic and fluctuate with hormonal changes just before and during the menses, which suggests a hormonal link that confirms the assumed gender-specific nature of chocolate cravings. Chocolate contains several biologically active constituents, all of which potentially cause abnormal behaviors and psychological sensations parallel to those of other addictive substances.[1]

Abstracted from the
Journal of the American Dietetic Association

Eating behavior is often controlled by environmental and mood variables. These include: the need to eat while "on the go" (in the car or on the commuter train), snacking to make a mundane task more enjoyable, the sociality of dining with friends, availability of forbidden foods, craving sweets, fatigue, irritability, boredom, depression, and skipping meals.[2]

Disease in general can be considered as a reaction to insults modified by individual susceptibility.

The drug [or food] abuser rarely realizes when he or she becomes an addict. The craving is irresistible, and anyone who has attempted to overcome a relatively mild form of drug dependency – like smoking – knows about those dark and impelling forces that slumber beneath the conscious level of our volitional selves.

When addiction sets in, that in and of itself becomes a pathological condition – with its own special characteristics and its own dynamics. Addiction is bound to develop if certain substances are administered in certain quantities over a certain period of time.

Lawrence D Dickey, MD,
in *Clincial Ecology*,
Charles C Thomas, publishers,
1976

THE HEART OF THIS PROGRAM . . .

At the heart of losing weight with the *California Calcium Countdown* is the belief that a major cause for the usual weight-loss dieting failure is the lack of knowledge about the role of cravings. A craving is defined as a fervent desire or longing to eat a particular food.[3] It represents one of the most common and intense experiences related to eating.[4] I am not referring to *psychological* dependence, but to a very real *physiological* addiction to foods that you should be avoiding. Foods, independent of chemical additives or contaminants, are our primary potential addictants.

The wrong food (even if it's a healthful or a low-calorie food or an improper dietary supplement), can disrupt normal metabolism. If you have a hidden allergy or intolerance to that food or supplement, it may promote fat storage and inhibit weight loss.[5] (A typical example of a health product that could activate hidden-allergy consequences is lecithin if the source of the lecithin is soy or egg, two common allergens.)[6]

FAST FOODS AND ADDICTIVE REACTIONS

Consumption of fast foods or processed foods, because of their high fat and/or sugar content, can trigger chemical reactions in your brain which can lead to overeating.

The biochemical changes caused by fat and sugar are comparable to the addictive reactions generated by taking drugs such as heroin and cocaine. That may be why it's no easy task to revert to a healthful diet after consuming foods containing these ingredients.[7]

Allergy and addiction are more closely related than you may think. Very compelling reasons demonstrate why we have so much trouble giving up the foods that cause subtle but ultimately debilitating allergic or sensitivity responses, and why these very foods are likely to be the foods we like best and consume most frequently.

We are all familiar with the syndrome of overeating carbohydrates to make ourselves feel better (particularly snack foods). This tendency to use certain foods as though they are drugs can also be seen in those who gain weight when exposed to stress, in women with premenstrual syndrome, in those suffering from "winter depression," and in people who are attempting to give up smoking.[8]

KNOWN WAY BACK WHEN

Food intolerance was noted by Hippocrates some time around 400 BC. In the early part of the twentieth century, we began to understand the physiology of immune reactions, but we had to wait four more decades for deep insight and clarification of the pathology of these reactions.[9]

Many people don't even know they have allergies. Unfortunately, the subject of food allergies has never assumed the importance that it is due. Part of the reason for this is that food allergies and food intolerance, although common, are difficult to diagnose and even more difficult to treat.[10] The interval between ingesting the offending food and the appearance of symptoms may vary widely from seconds to several days.

Experts consider food sensitivities to be the most commonly undiagnosed illness in medicine.[11]

Recently, food sensitivities have been implicated in conditions as varied as Attention Deficit Disorder (ADD), diarrhea, rheumatoid arthritis, diabetes, heart disease, peptic ulcers, celiac disease, multiple sclerosis, thyroiditis, psoriasis, asthma, and mental problems (including depression and schizophrenia).

Our concern here, of course, is that allergies and food sensitivities can cause weight gain. In short, consuming food allergens stimulates the release of insulin, which causes hypoglycemia (low blood sugar). This, in turn, usually results in extreme hunger – a feeling that you must eat NOW. Although any food can spark hypoglycemia, amino acids, sugars and carbohydrates (breads and pasta) are common offenders.[12]

ALLERGY VS SENSITIVITY: UNDERSTANDING THE DIFFERENCES

What are the differences between food allergy and food sensitivity? And just how does addiction play out in terms of failed attempts at dieting? Sometimes, the vocabulary is used interchangeably. Following are basic definitions.

Allergies. Allergies are a very common problem, affecting at least 2 out of every 10 Americans, and possibly more, depending on how the term is defined. People who have allergies have hyper-alert immune systems that overreact to a substance in the environment. This substance is called an allergen. Exposure to a substance that is normally harmless (such as pollen) causes the immune system to respond as if the substance is harmful.

If the allergen is in the air, the allergic response will occur in your eyes, nose, and lungs. If the allergen is ingested, the allergic reaction will present itself in your mouth, stomach, and intestines. Sometimes enough chemicals are released during an allergic response to cause a disruption throughout your body, such as hives, decreased blood pressure, shock, or loss of consciousness. This severe type of allergic reaction is called anaphylaxis and it can be life-threatening.

Allergy can affect different parts of the ears. Before having tubes placed in your child's ears, check their diets and their allergies.[13]

Allergies to peanuts are responsible for nearly 100 deaths and 15,000 visits to emergency rooms – about half the deaths and emergency room visits caused by *all* food allergies – each year.

Prevalence of peanut allergy in children doubled over a five-year period, according to a study published in the December 2003 issue of the *Journal of Allergy and Clinical Immunology*.

Food Allergies. Oops! Your immune system blundered! A food allergy occurs when your body mistakes an ingredient in food – usually a protein – as threatening, and creates a defense system (antibodies) to fight it. Allergy symptoms develop when the antibodies are battling the "invading" food, which your body interprets as an enemy.

Symptoms can include a rash or hives, nausea, stomach pain, diarrhea, itchy skin, shortness of breath, chest pain, swelling of the airways to the lungs, rapid pulse, and anaphylaxis.

Food Intolerance (also referred to as Food Sensitivity). Food intolerance is a *digestive system* response rather than an immune response. It occurs when something in food irritates your digestive system or when you are unable to properly digest or break down the food. Intolerance to lactose, found in milk and milk products, is a common food intolerance.

Lactose Intolerance

Most of us are technically lactose-intolerant to some degree because we stop manufacturing an enzyme (called lactase) some time between early childhood and adolescence. As we approach teen years, we have a diminished capacity to break down milk sugar.

There's nothing surprising about our loss of this ability to metabolize milk sugar. Very few, if any, of the world's indigenous populations have access to any significant amount of milk in their diet other than human milk in early childhood.

The majority of the world's population – excluding northern European ethnic groups (Nordic, Germanic, Anglo-Saxon) and isolated populations in Africa and the Indian subcontinent – has primary lactase deficiency.[14] The same is true of *all* mammals. Animals do not consume milk after weaning, nor do they ever consume the milk of another species.

We used to think that those individuals who didn't produce lactase in adulthood had abnormal digestive processes. Now we consider those who *do* produce lactase beyond childhood as the aberrant ones, having genetic malfunctions.[15]

Symptoms of lactose intolerance can range from mild to extremely painful.

Food reactions are more common than food allergies, and are more frequent than most people realize.[16] Think about it: How often have you had an unpleasant reaction to something you ate? You may have very specific food intolerances, such as with lactose intolerance.

Nonspecific food reactions may occur because of additives in certain foods, because of food rancidity, or because your immune system is just not up to par at a particular time. The backlash can be nausea, stomach pain, gas, cramps or bloating, vomiting, heartburn, diarrhea, headaches, irritability or nervousness.[17]

Food allergies can be triggered by even a small amount of the food in question and can occur every time that particular food is consumed. But food intolerances are usually dose- and frequency-related. The more often you swallow the culprit and the greater the quantity, the more likely you are to have an adverse reaction.

If you have an unpleasant symptom following a meal (even fatigue, a common reaction), it is most likely intolerance rather than allergy. (Remember, intolerance or sensitivity is not the same as the immune response of an allergy.) But be aware that *any* food consumed in excessive quantity can cause digestive symptoms. This stems from a different causative factor than allergy or sensitivity.[18] (Think of all those times you've found yourself saying "I can't believe I ate the whole thing!")

Many factors may contribute to food intolerance. In some cases, as with lactose intolerance, you are missing the enzymes necessary to properly digest the offending food. Also common are intolerances to chemical ingredients added to food to provide color (red and yellow dyes), enhance taste (MSG), and protect against the growth of bacteria (sprays on vegetables in salad bars).

Sulfites may be added to foods to prevent the growth of mold, and they are a source of intolerance for many (especially those with respiratory problems). I have an intolerance to both sulfites and to the chemicals in the papers that emerge from my office printer. Sulfites appear to close my throat; the paper chemicals cause me to sneeze about a dozen or more times.

However, taking the buffered C and mineral formula referred to earlier and described in detail in chapter seven, causes the throat-closing and the sneezing to stop instantly.

Now that I take this formula regularly, the symptoms rarely occur.

If you are in good health nutritionally, you have a better chance of having symptom-free adaptations to foods that would otherwise cause reactions. But it is not uncommon for symptom-free adaptation to change to *maladapted* responses during and following infections, especially viral infections.[19] For example, you may be more susceptible to unpleasant reactions to Salmonella or E coli exposure when your health is below par, just as a high amount of vitamin C that would normally cause stomach upset can be well tolerated when you have certain illnesses.

In summary, *allergy* should be distinguished from the broader term *food intolerance.*

Food intolerance may be defined as a reproducible adverse reaction to the ingestion of a food or to any of its components, ie, proteins, carbohydrates, fats, and additives, and which includes toxic, metabolic, and allergic reactions.

Food allergy, by contrast, may be defined as an adverse clinical reaction to a specific food component that is immunologically mediated.[20]

FOOD SENSITIVITIES
AND THE AMERICAN DIET

According to the Us Department of Agriculture, these are the foods to which Americnas are most sensitive:

~ whole cow's milk
~ 2% cow's milk
~ processed American cheese
~ bread and rolls (made from processed wheat)
~ wheat flour (found in many foods, like soups and cereals)
~ refined sugar (which comprise 15% to 21% of all calories)
~ soft drinks
~ ground beef

It is interesting to note that these are the foods consumed by Americans more than any other foods.

TRACKING DOWN YOUR OWN FOOD CULPRIT

The management of a food allergy begins with recognizing the responsible allergens. If you are really serious about identifying your specific food problems, you need to stop eating your favorite foods (the ones you crave, the ones you just can't do without) for *four full days*. If you are sensitive to this food or foods, you will go through actual withdrawal, just as surely as if you were quitting smoking or stopping your caffeine consumption.

The success of this elimination diet depends on several factors. You need to correctly identify the food involved and you must maintain a diet completely free of all forms of that possible offending food. In addition, no other factors should provoke similar symptoms during that time. Unless all these conditions are met, your test will fall short of being accurate.[21]

Finding the origin of your food problem this way may appear to be time-consuming and annoying. But it could be easier than resisting a hot-fudge sundae. You may be cranky; you may have trouble sleeping; you may have an ongoing headache; you may feel depressed or unusually tired. An insatiable hunger is a common withdrawal symptom.[22] If this is the problem food, you will begin to feel better in about ten days to two weeks. At that time, if you reintroduce the food, your symptoms may return worse than ever, and this is the signal that this is NOT the food for you. The good news is that once the incriminated food or foods are avoided and/or spared, there is a marked reduction in the hunger pangs. (Better news is that you may be able to avert the problem with the buffered C/mineral formula, explained in detail in chapter seven.)

Reducing the intake of these foods instead of avoiding them not only accentuates the clinical features of food addiction, but virtually precludes following such a diet. Far more successful is the identification and avoidance of the fallen-angel foods.

FOUR-DAY PASS-THROUGH

The four-day challenge test is nothing new. Hippocrates reported in his writings the knowledge that if a food is avoided for as much as four days, a reexposure to that food might create a severe reaction in certain people. It seems to take at least that many days for any food or chemical to be entirely eliminated from the human system – whether you are living now or lived 2500 years ago![23]

Keep in mind that the foods that usually cause the most problems are the ones you eat most frequently. Again, among the foods causing difficulty are milk (and milk products), wheat (including bread, muffins, donuts, cookies, pizza, pie crust, etc.) and sugar. Soy, corn, yeast, coffee, commercial eggs and citrus are also high on the list. Although any food may cause an allergic reaction, only a few foods account for 90 percent of such reactions. In children, these foods are eggs, milk, peanuts, soy, and wheat. (If the average American emptied the fridge of all these potentially allergenic foods, chances are there would be nothing left but the light bulb.)

Although milk allergy is noted in adults, allergies to nuts, peanuts, seafood and eggs are more common. This is in contrast to cow's milk allergy in children, which, during infancy, is one of the most common food allergies. However, the allergy to milk may be one of two forms: one that is transient and outgrown after childhood; another remains a problem for life.[24]

MILK PROBLEM FROM MOM

The presence of food allergy at birth has been attributed to exposure in the fetal stage. In other words, the baby is the recipient of the allergenic substance through Mom's diet. But it doesn't explain why milk allergy, the most common food sensitivity, is often present at birth in infants born of mothers who never take milk in any form.[25] [This may indicate hidden casein, the protein in milk that could be the trouble-maker in processed foods.]

FOOD ON THE BRAIN

Sadly, the foods you crave do more than undermine your health. As described, they can cause addictions akin to and severe as those experienced with alcohol, drugs, or tobacco, and even come with unpleasant withdrawal symptoms. *Why oh why do we crave the foods that do us in?*

The reason you feel so gratified when you consume such foods is that they initiate pleasure-inducing chemicals secreted by your adrenal glands and by your brain.

And, just as with alcohol, recreational drugs, or tobacco, these foods make you feel "high."

Chemicals in milk and wheat have been shown to cause opiates to be released from your brain. Opiates are the brain's built-in *feeling-on-top-of-the-world morphine-like substances*. The opioids seem to influence food palatability, and they appear to be released when you eat foods rich in sugar and fat.[26] Since they make you feel so terrific, you want more of these foods. What an unfortunate phenomenon, no doubt programmed before the advent of processed foods. This flurry of brain function may be experienced by most grade school children on a daily basis when they come home to milk and cookies.

The major point is that food cravings are not like normal hunger. They are responsible for overeating, too often on fattening food. And they lead to *addiction* to the very foods you crave.

Most sensitive people are likely to eat a very monotonous diet of just a few foods, tending to go from one damaging food to the next, usually selected from the short list of foods on the chart on page 53. A monotonous diet is frequently also an addictive diet.

Michael Rosenbaum, MD, who heads a very successful medical clinic in Corte Madera, California, states:

> **Food sensitivities can cause your body to retain both water and fat.** Food allergies need to be accounted for and dealt with when planning a sensible weight management program. In my experience, when a patient hits a plateau and cannot lose weight, I will institute a food rotation diet. It almost never fails to quickly shed those stubborn pounds.

Rosenbaum pinpointed the very reason all these popular food-fad diets fail.

The first physician to publish a book titled *Calories Don't Count* was actually jailed for promoting concepts contrary to current medical opinion of the time. We now know that counting calories has done little, if anything, to help this country's scale readings from zooming so high.

COUNT CARBS, NOT CALORIES

DR. HERMAN TALLER claimed in his 1961 book *Calories Don't Count* that a high-fat, high-protein, low-carbohydrate diet was the ticket to a healthier, leaner life. Taller, a Brooklyn, New York, obstetrician-gynecologist, was, like Dr Atkins, following in the low-carb footsteps of William Banting and Alfred Pennington. According to reports, the medical community was out to get him for the *calories don't count* concept. In 1967 he was accused of fraud by the Food and Drug Administration for claiming his safflower capsules would help reduce body fat. (Even this concept has validity today. A small amount of polyunsaturated oil can help fat reduction. A few slices of avocado, however, are a better way to go than ingesting a potentially rancid vegetable oil.)

THE SEROTONIN CONNECTION

Carbohydrate craving is considered the consequence of a decrease of serotonin, the neurotransmitter mentioned in the first chapter. When the medical community tried to control serotonin with the use of drugs, it was eventually discovered that a serious side effect resulted – one that adversely affected the heart.[27] This brought us back to square one.

Cells that are normally in charge of the release of serotonin are usually controlled by food intake. But serotonin release is also involved in such functions as sleep onset, pain sensitivity, blood pressure regulation, and control of mood. This is why many people learn to overeat carbohydrates (particularly snack foods like potato chips or pastries, which are rich in carbohydrates and fat) to make themselves feel better.[28]

CRAVERS TAKE NOTE

~ Low-calorie breakfasts lead to increased hunger and cravings during the morning and at lunch compared with those who take a high-energy breakfast. A low-energy breakfast fails to generate the satiety signals induced by a breakfast of about 500 calories.[29] It's the low-calorie breakfast eaters who clock-watch for the coffee break.

~ Craving for a particular food increases after exposure to the smell and thought of that food. You can see how cues increase craving.[30]

~ Food cravings are more common among women and are frequently associated with specific types of foods, including chocolate and foods high in both sugar and fat.[31] This is true for Americans, but not necessarily for other cultures, which argues against a physiological basis for chocolate craving.[32]

~ Cravers, especially women, are more frequently concerned about their weight than noncravers. Energy intake for snacks is higher in cravers. Less than 40 percent of cravers report being hungry when they experience cravings. Food craving episodes are also strongly associated with mood.[33]

~ A desire for *more* occurs during, rather than preceding, an eating episode, and is experienced when the eater attempts to limit consumption before the appetite for the food has been satisfied. This is common with chocolate consumption.[34]

~ If you have allergies and you are pregnant, cesarean delivery increases your child's chances of subsequent food allergy.[35]

~ Women with a higher body mass report more consistent cravings for salty foods. But chocolate and ice cream are still highest on the craving list, followed by fatty foods, and spicy foods and sweets.[36]

~ In overweight people, evidence points to a defect in the control of fat intake. In these people, dietary fat exerts only a weak action on satiety; it fails to generate strong responses in the mechanisms of the satiety cascade.[37]

~ Cravings tend to occur late in the afternoon and early evening.[38]

~ After a protein-rich meal, craving for sweet, carbohydrate-rich foods is significantly higher than after a carbohydrate and mixed meal.[39]

~ Studies report carbohydrate cravings in the premenstrual phase, particularly in women with premenstrual syndrome, and is often associated with low serotonin activity.[40]

This is the part of the menstrual cycle surrounding the onset of menstruation, a time when progesterone is low. Increasing progesterone levels at this time, however, does not decrease chocolate or sweets craving.[41]

~ Craving for chocolate or other foods may be an expression of a strong appetite elicited by hunger that has been acquired by repeated experience of eating the craved food when hungry.[42]

Although chocolate is a food which provides pleasure, for those who consider intake of this food to be excessive, any pleasure experienced is short-lived and accompanied by feelings of guilt.[43]

~ Carbohydrate cravers report feeling distressed prior to their cravings and satisfied, happy/good and relaxed following carbohydrate consumption. Protein cravers report feeling anxious or hungry prior to their cravings and happy, normal, bored, and energetic following protein-rich food consumption.[44]

~ Craving sweets is negatively associated with hunger and is not associated with meal skipping.[45]

~ Nervousness, craving, insomnia, and irritability are associated with withdrawal from excessive carrot eating. The basis for this is believed to be beta-carotene, found in carrots. Does carrot eating, an aggressively oral activity, merely act as a behavioral substitute for smoking? Or does beta-carotene contain a chemical element that replicates the addictive component of nicotine?

Further study of this unusual but intriguing addiction may reveal more about the basis of *all* addictions, with particular implications for the cessation of cigarette smoking.[46]

~ Breathing in the vapors of black pepper essential oil can curtail cigarette craving during withdrawal of nicotine.[47]

TO EACH HIS OWN

Lucretius, who lived in the first century BC, had the insight to see that intolerance is an individual peculiarity entirely unrelated to the nature of food. We are all familiar with his widely quoted comment, "What is food to one may be fierce poison to others."[48]

Why hasn't our medical community been paying attention to the interrelationship between cravings and our serious overweight problem? Simple! There is a natural lapse of time between the appearances of a first study – however controlled, objective, double-blinded or prestigious – to the time the information is medically accepted and becomes touted as common knowledge. When ideas have been around for a long time, they are rarely questioned. As new research creates an upheaval of fixed beliefs, we all (including our doctors) have difficulty accepting the change.

~~~~~

A recent issue of our government's *Morbidity and Mortality Weekly Report* confirms that we have made little headway against the problem of overweight.[49] Worse, we have come to accept irregularities as normal. Suboptimal nutrition is the rule, not the exception. It's of interest to conjecture what we would be like if we all had abundant calcium and an array of all the other good-health nutrients. What if our collective nutrition could be at a level of excellence? What if we didn't have any sensitivities, or if our cravings were only for wholesome foods? What if only wholesome foods were widely available? Read on for an intriguing answer to these questions.

Chapter Four

EXPANDING PROBLEM;
GETTING WORSE

THE DENTIST WHO TRAVELED THE WORLD

Say "ah"! What Dr. Weston Price saw in the mouths of his patients back in the 1930s was not too different from what yur dentist would see today: *deformed arches, crooked teeth, crowded teeth, cavities.* Then, as now, patients were suffering from increasing degenerative and chronic diseases. Those with the worst teeth were also the primary contenders for tuberculosis – one of the most common infectious diseases of that time. (In 1937, when I was twelve, I had a dozen cavities; I had contracted diphtheria by age six.)

So what was causing these health problems? Was it stress? Poor diet? Bad air? Not enough water? Lack of exercise? Or perhaps some unknown factor related to civilized societies?

Determined to find answers, Price began an unusual odyssey – one with results so powerful, it should have changed the way people thought about health *and* disease. Unfortunately, it had little impact on our lifestyles or health statistics.

Price and his wife packed their bags, and off they went to remote locations around the globe, where he studied communities of people who were remarkably free of disease – and, by the way, were not overweight – a trend already well underway in the US even back then!

Over a period of nine years, Price visited fourteen different groups of native peoples, from the islands of the Scottish Hebrides to the Swiss Alps, from Polynesia to the Andes Mountains in Peru. This was no easy task in the days before jet airplanes, but Weston Price's commitment to seek answers was boundless

When Price told these far-flung patients to open their mouths, what he discovered was quite another story. He saw glowing health, reflected in normal gum tissue and a paucity of cavities. He observed strong bone structure and almost no degenerative diseases.

This was true despite sometimes harsh living conditions – such as those endured by Eskimos living above the Arctic Circle or Peruvian natives high in the Andes. When he did find a few unhealthy native cultures, usually they were suffering from health problems related to food shortages or drought.

The diets of the people Price visited were widely diverse, but he confirmed certain similarities common to most of the cultures. *The foods eaten were generally fresh, often raw, and, of course, completely natural and organic.* Price also noticed that almost all the groups ate some fermented foods every day, rich in digestive enzymes and vitamin K.

When he analyzed food samples, Price learned that they contained many times the nutrients found in the American diet, including about *four* **times the amount of calcium**. To Price, this explained not only the good health, but also the *longevity* of these various peoples.

Although some may have died young due to dangerous or life-threatening living conditions, those who did survive remained healthy and strong well into their golden years.

At the same time, those who converted to new diets (that is, meals consisting mostly of canned goods, white flour products, and other processed foods) began to get the kind of diseases common to us "civilized" folk. As a dentist, Price took special note of the large increase in dental problems in the modernized groups, where dental cavities increased by a factor of ten or more.[1] (To learn more about the work of Dr. Price and the foundation that continues his work, see Appendix B.)

One aspect of Weston Price's observations that we in the US should not ignore is childbirth risk. Our current birth morbidity and mortality statistics are shamefully low. Most of the indigenous tribes or villages visited by Price understood the importance of prenatal nutrition.

Choice foods were given to both pregnant and lactating women, and these foods were especially high in calcium.

~ In one of Africa's rural districts, primitive Masai girls were instructed to delay marriage until the time of the year that the cows ate young grass, as the milk these cows produced was of a superior quality. After six months of the girls consuming this high-nutrient food, marriage was allowed.[2] Whole milk, of course, is high in calcium, with 300 mg per cup. Technology has taught us that young green grasses are also especially high in calcium, so chances are that this milk had an even *higher calcium* content. Nor, of course, was this milk pasteurized, a process that significantly reduces calcium.

~ In the Fiji Islands two young men were assigned the task of doing the "marketplace" shopping for a pregnant woman: It was their daily job to obtain from the sea a particular kind of crab that was extraordinarily rich in nutrients.[3]

Crabs are always included on lists of high-calcium foods!

~ Among Eskimos, fish eggs were eaten by childbearing women. Coastal Indians in Peru also knew this great secret.[4] (Fish roe are among the most healthful foods on our planet. Needless to say, they have a high **calcium** content.)

~ Expectant mothers of several African tribes depended on a form of red millet for their **calcium** intake. This same cereal was used in Peru by nursing mothers as an encouragement for milk flow.[5]

This particular red millet has a calcium rating five to ten times higher than other cereals.

It's also amazing that such distant cultures would follow the same dietary customs – but as is so often the case, those who live closer to nature understand its wisdom much better than those of us lost in the "modern" world.

Oh . . . and did I already mention that the healthy people Weston Price encountered were not overweight?

"THE MILK OF THE OCEAN"

Are Weston Price's assumptions about calcium supported by modern research? The authors of *The Okinawa Program* think so. They report studies on the health and longevity of the people of Okinawa, a chain of small tropical islands in southern Japan. There is strong evidence that the natives of Okinawa are the longest-living people in the world today, with *many* among them celebrating birthdays well into their nineties, and longer.[6] In fact, Okinawa has the highest percentage of 100-year olds in the world.

What is of special interest in Okinawa is the quantity of (you guessed it!) *calcium* and magnesium found in the island drinking water. Because these islands are comprised of coral reefs, the decaying coral, which is high in calcium and other minerals, is present in the spring water. (Later I discuss *coral calcium*, its potential value and why it should not be dismissed despite blatant over-promotion.)

The Okinawa researchers theorize that the longevity and low incidence of degenerative diseases observed in these islanders are consistent with the high levels of calcium, magnesium and trace minerals found in their drinking water, along with their high vitamin D levels due to long hours in the bright sunshine.

People in Okinawa today present a profile of health that is strikingly similar to those studied by Weston Price.

Indeed, high levels of calcium, magnesium and trace minerals in drinking water seem to be a common factor among long-living peoples everywhere. Many centenarians reside in mountainous regions, like the Andes or the Caucasus, and drink water from melting glaciers, water that is often whitish in tint because of dissolved calcium and other minerals. This is the "milk of the mountains" – or, in Okinawa, the "milk of the ocean."

Like the peoples Price visited, the healthy Okinawans had a very low incidence of obesity.

CALCIUM AND THE CAVEMEN

Studies by Dr. Robert Heaney, a renowned calcium researcher, adds even more credibility to the work of Dr. Price and *The Okinawa Program* scientists.

Heaney believes that calcium was much more prevalent in our very early food supply. The calcium intake of many Stone Age adults is estimated to have been three-to-five times the calcium intake of modern US adults, or from 2,000 to 3,000 milligrams per day. Heaney suggests that the body's calcium regulatory mechanism has evolved over time as a result of greater availability of calcium. At high levels, calcium is *not* a quick-picker-upper, as discussed in chapter two. The more calcium ingested, the less absorbed.[7]

At the other end of the scale, however, the smaller the intake of calcium – the smaller the dietary supply – the more efficient the absorption. Nature has its checks and balances.

So while the general trend has been the consumption of less calcium than our distant ancestors ate, and our greater intake of calcium antagonists (phosphorus in particular), our bodies have retained the adaptive mechanisms better suited to prehistoric calcium consumption.

According to Heaney, this may play a role in promoting ***those excess pounds***. The problem might be reversed by improving our intake of calcium, magnesium and vitamin D in supplemental form.[8] This will be discussed in detail in chapter seven.

A very important concept to keep in mind is that diets high in phosphorus initiate results similar to calcium deficiency.

Heany explains the consequences this way: Adequate calcium is a signal to fat tissue that your body is well nourished. This indicator tells your body that it no longer needs to store fat, but can burn it. Fat storage is reversed and fat burning is increased.

In test animals on a low-calcium diet, an enzyme increases fat *deposition* by 2.6 times. But with high dietary calcium, fat *burning* is boosted by 3.4 to 5.2 times. The increased burning of fat causes the elevations in body temperature – either directly, or by stimulating a special protein that leads to temperature elevation due to metabolism.[9]

According to the National Institutes of Health, *calcium intake up to about 2,000 milligrams a day in supplemental form appears to be safe in most individuals.*[10]

S. Boyd Eaton, a physician also known for his studies on Paleolithic diets, analyzed more than one hundred plant foods consumed by tribes of hunter-gatherers. Eaton's results support the notion that high levels of calcium intake are desirable because our physiologies developed this way over generations. Wild vegetable foods average about 130 milligrams of calcium per 100-gram portions. (100 grams is somewhat equal to an amount of food the size of your fist, a common standard in food comparisons.)

Late Paleolithic people were eating about 1,460 grams of such food each day, so plant foods would have produced over 1,800 milligrams of calcium while the meat they ate would have supplied another 100 milligrams. Gnawing on bones from fowl (as I remember my grandmother doing) or from small mammals might have substantially increased the amount of calcium ingested.

Eaton confirms that the nutritional requirements of contemporary humans were almost certainly established over eons of evolutionary experience and the best available evidence indicates that this evolution occurred in a high-calcium nutritional environment. The exercise and dietary patterns of humans living at the end of the Stone Age can be considered natural paradigms: Calcium intake was *twice* what it is for contemporary humans. Requirements for physical exertion were also much greater. And again, there were no processed foods or the kind of calcium antagonists we encounter today. Bone remains from that period suggest that Stone Agers developed a greater peak bone mass and experienced less age-related bone loss than do humans today.[11]

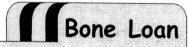

Bone Loan

THE BONE "LOAN"

Primitive human diets had very high calcium nutrient densities. Human physiology was optimized to prevent excessive intakes. When calcium deficient, the skeleton served as a reserve for calcium by increasing bony resorption [sending calcium back into the blood from the bone]. When food supplies were plentiful, this skeletal "loan" was repaid. In contrast, agricultural societies have diets with low calcium densities because they are based on seed foods, which have the lowest calcium content of all the plant parts.

Modern humans, faced with lower calcium intake [and battling against calcium antagonists], must adapt continuously, dealing with *calcium* shortage by using mechanisms evolved for *food* shortage – by withdrawing calcium from the skeletal reserves (ie, decreasing bone mass).[12]

One consequence is that certain hormones rise progressively with age. Three years of calcium supplementation reduces these hormonal substances to levels similar to those of young adult normal values, but never *below* normal.[13]

Adapted from the *American Journal of Clinical Nutrition* and the *Journal of Clinical Endocrinology and Metabolism*.

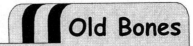

THE BONES IN THE CHURCH: A PEAK INTO THE PAST

The incidence of osteoporotic hip fractures has been increasing faster than the rate expected if it were adjusted for life expectancy. The restoration of a London church, during which bone fragments dating from 1729 to 1852 were recovered, provided a unique opportunity to compare the occurrence of historical bone loss with that of present-day women.

Women today suffer far greater bone loss than they did two centuries ago, both pre- and postmenopausally. Researchers saw the typical decline in premenopausal bone density in present-day women but found no significant loss in the preserved samples. This suggests that a 70-year-old woman today would have a lower bone density than would a 70-year-old woman who lived two centuries ago.[14] This should set you thinking!

Excerpted from *Hormone Replacement Therapy: Yes or No, How to Make an Informed Decision* Betty Kamen, Nutrition Encounter, 2002.

A VITAMIN D MYSTERY

People of European ancestry represent an interesting example of metabolic diversity. White-skinned people metabolize vitamin D from sunshine very differently than those with darker skins. Darker-skinned people need longer exposure to sunshine to manufacture vitamin D, and this has a direct effect on calcium metabolism because vitamin D is critical for the absorption and utilization of calcium.

Despite this physiological difference, blacks have denser bones than do whites. The fact that blacks have the slowest rate of bone loss adds to the metabolic puzzle, since vitamin D is crucial to bone-health pathways, and as mentioned, increased skin pigmentation greatly reduces the manufacture of vitamin D from sun exposure. It takes six times the dose of standard ultraviolet rays to increase circulating vitamin D in blacks to concentrations similar to those recorded in white people.[15]

To further confuse the issue, black adults have less osteoporosis, but black children have a higher incidence of rickets [a deficiency disease affecting skeletal growth].[16] So what's going on?

UNDERSTANDING THE DISEASE PROCESS

Since the time of Hippocrates (460–377 BC), and even before, we have had scientists who understood the relationship between the foods we ate and our health status. Decades ago, I was fortunate enough to benefit from the advice of one such physician, Dr. George Congram of Hicksville, Long Island, NY. Congram's teachings and those of his colleagues are just now beginning to be understood and acknowledged. He taught me to sprout, to juice vegetables, to detoxify, to scrape the white pulp of organic oranges and grapefruits for their high bioflavonoid content (this predates the availability of bioflavonoids from a bottle), and the importance of taking the right kind of supplements, including **calcium, magnesium and vitamin D.**

Another innovator with whom I interacted was endocrinologist Harold Rosenberg of New York City. Rosenberg was among the first to recognize the causes and cures of hypoglycemia (low blood sugar) in this country. (The condition was initially described by the incarcerated physicians in the Warsaw Ghetto during World War II, and published in a compelling book years later called *The Hunger Disease.*) Because of his expertise in this field of work, Rosenberg was able to pinpoint with great accuracy the blood sugar level of his patients by the responses he saw in their veins when he drew blood. His suppositions were always on target, confirmed by laboratory testing. He was also a great believer in the importance of calcium, vitamin D and other special nutrients as supplements. Patients who followed the suggested regimens of these innovative doctors were not overweight. (How is that for a plus?)

Dr. Carl Reich of Calgary, Alberta, was another doctor who used substantial doses of vitamin D more than half a century ago. He perceived that the lack of vitamin D – whether caused by deficits in food, supplements, or sunlight – was a major problem of our age. Fifty years later, on October 10, 2003, medical experts at the National Institutes of Health talked about a "new" health epidemic: *the lack of vitamin D.*[17]

Congram, Rosenberg and Reich were able to test their theories over many years. Every day, they saw proof that calcium, magnesium and vitamin D, and other key nutrients, were helpful factors in curing disease. The positive results were generally quick and dramatic, helping to confirm their convictions.

The lack of calcium, magnesium, and vitamin D has been implicated in a very large number of disorders and diseases, including osteoporosis, high blood pressure, diabetes, arthritis and **obesity**. It may come as a surprise that the association between many health challenges and particular nutrient inadequacies was not generally recognized up until the 1950s. Nor was the correlation between hypoglycemia, diet and weight problems. As recently as the early 1980s, I was reprimanded by the American Medical Association for suggesting that a deficiency of folic acid could be the cause of serious birth anomalies.[18] Twenty years later, this fact is common knowledge.

A TEAM PLAYER

How can the calcium coursing through your blood perform all those duties, cited earlier, if there isn't enough to go around? The answer is *it can't*. Not only do our bones serve as a backup system, but calcium's alliance with other nutrients is also critical. Examples of calcium's nutrient codependence follow.

~ Enough vitamin D is needed to help absorb calcium from your digestive system and to help regulate its many functions.

~ Magnesium works in tandem with calcium in your muscles, nerves and body tissues, especially in the regulation of heart and muscle contraction and nerve conduction. It also helps to control the passage of nutrients into your cells and supports the excretion of wastes. Without magnesium, too much calcium may build up in your cells, which can lead to a number of serious disorders. (Heart patients, take note.)

~ Phosphorus works with calcium to encourage strength and rigidity of bones.

~ Vitamins C and K, along with calcium, activate proteins that encourage bone formation.[19]

See chapter seven for more associations.

SYNDROME X

Although it sounds like it's straight out of a B movie, *Syndrome X* (also referred to as *Metabolic Syndrome*) has become a common medical term.

A WAIST IS A TERRIBLE THING TO MIND

If you have a relatively large waist and an excess of fats in your blood you are more likely to be at risk for Syndrome X. The threshold value for waist size is about 38 inches in men and about 45 inches in women.

The number of people with waist sizes above the threshold levels increases with age, going from 6 percent between ages 18–24 to 43 percent between 44–74. What is going on is a decreased capacity to get rid of fat fuels; you store them instead. The problem is that you begin to store fat in non-fat tissue, such as your liver and skeletal tissue. Now other problems (like insulin resistance, explained below), high blood pressure, and glucose in-tolerance) arise.[20]

For most people, the root causes of this syndrome are improper nutrition, inadequate physical activity, and increases in weight. Too many refined carbohydrates (sweets and baked goods) contribute to the syndrome.[21] The cornerstones of treatment are weight loss and appropriate levels of physical activity. (So what else is new? How many times have we heard this before?)

The term *Syndrome X* was coined by Stanford University endocrinologist Gerald Reaven in 1988 to describe a group of symptoms that include high blood pressure, an excess of insulin in the blood, and **obesity**. This trilogy of symptoms can lead to serious diseases such as diabetes, high blood pressure and certain heart problems.[22]

That same year, my book, *The Chromium Connection: A Lesson in Nutrition*, was published. I was impressed enough with the first presentation of information about Syndrome X to include it in my chapter on heart health. It took more than a decade for the term to become more commonly associated with the syndrome of symptoms it described.

Why should we care about Syndrome X? Because its victims gain weight easily and have a difficult time losing it. Worse, it imposes substantial risk for type 2 diabetes and premature coronary heart disease. And – are you ready for this? – a study published in the *Journal of the American Medical Association* advises that a staggering *fifty million people* have the syndrome in the US – with many more at risk![23]

Excess body weight is a symptom, not a cause. Again, inadequate calcium and magnesium may play a significant role. If you are interested in how this comes about, read on. If not, skip down to the heading: CALCIUM AND MAGNESIUM TO THE RESCUE.

AVOIDING (THE) IRS

Don't call your accountant – it's not what you think! IRS stands for *insulin resistance syndrome*, which may translate to overweight, little physical activity, smoking, high cholesterol levels, inappropriate diet, and/or a high risk of hypertension, cardiovascular disease and stroke. Another word creeping into medical jargon is *diabesity*, a term combining obesity and type II diabetes.[24]

Insulin resistance refers to a condition in which insulin is present to escort glucose to cells, but the cells refuse to admit the glucose. This is serious because glucose is our cell's source of fuel, or energy.

Receptor sites are receivers on the surfaces of our cells that allow cells to combine with materials traveling through our blood. Insulin receptors are like magnets – they are designed to attract the hormone insulin, and pull it into our cells. This is the way insulin regulates the amount of glucose (blood sugar) in the bloodstream. Receptor sites have also been likened to pieces of a jigsaw puzzle, with the appropriate molecule fitting perfectly into the appropriate receptor, and ONLY into that single molecule. (Incredible, when you think of the trillions of cells in your body.)

But your cells sometimes put up a barrier, and refuse to pick up the insulin they require. According to a study reported in the *American Journal of Clinical Nutrition* on food intake and body weight, this reaction is particularly true of muscle, liver, brain, and *adipose* [fatty] tissue. [25]

Here's what happens when things don't work as nature intended: An overload of refined carbohydrates floods your blood with glucose, which then accumulates in your bloodstream instead of entering your cells. Insulin-resistant muscle and liver cells both reduce energy reserves, and inertia is the result. In the case of the brain, thinking capacity suffers. And adipose tissue? Here comes the overweight component. What a triad! You've eaten those donuts, and now you're lethargic, dull, *and* overweight. And each of the consequences has an impact on the others.

Insulin resistance is a well-known occurrence among those who are overweight.[26] The **"Keep Out"** sign posted by your cells causes the insulin level in your blood to rise. High insulin levels can eventually lead to heart disease and diabetes. In 1989, the headline of a chilling article in *New England Journal of Medicine* was titled, "Insulin Resistance: A Secret Killer?"[27]

To add insult to injury, because insulin resistance is responsible for excess glucose *remaining* in your blood, your body now tries to reduce the amount of glucose by stimulating your pancreas to produce *more* insulin. Pretty soon your blood is brimming over with insulin. Some of the glucose may be converted to precursors of fats called triglycerides, which eventually become incorporated into fatty tissue.[28] And what you don't need now is more fat tissue![29]

Insulin has a profound effect on your appetite-regulating gland. As you eat and your blood glucose levels rise, your pancreas secretes insulin to take care of the newly arrived glucose. And as your insulin levels increase, your *appestat* is affected, and your hunger is appeased.[30] That's the way it *should* work.

Your appestat? Yes! Lying near the underside of your brain, just about in the center of your head, is your hypothalamus (Greek for *under the inner room*). Not much bigger than a small prune, this incredible, but seemingly trivial mass of cells acts as the command post for your brain. It's the message center that maintains equilibrium and informs other regions of your brain of their duties.

A portion of your hypothalamus is called the *satiety* center, or *appestat.* The appestat controls your appetite by communicating with your brain.[31] Did you know that you don't have the sensation of hunger until your hypothalamus sends a hunger signal to your brain?

The final demand is: FEED ME NOW!

Okay, so you eat and you feel satisfied. Your appestat is responsive to insulin levels, not to the quantity of food intake. These are good blueprints for control – if only they functioned with efficiency all the time. Here's the rub: Insulin resistance leads to a false perception of the inadequacy of food, resulting in overeating.[32] You may have plenty of insulin, but if your cell receptors can't recognize and utilize any of it, you just go on packing it away. (And all this time you thought you were "pigging out" because of lack of will power. Isn't it reassuring to know that's not an accurate picture?)

HUNGRY? IT MIGHT BE CHEMICAL

When the behavior-regulating neurotransmitter, serotonin, is out of order, it can cause uncurbed binge-eating. The result? Excessive consumption of refined carbohydrates, and/or cravings for sweets.[33]

Serotonin is made in your brain from tryptophan, an amino acid present in most foods. But tryptophan needs insulin to get into your brain.[34] Normally, a high carbohydrate meal stimulates insulin secretion, which enhances tryptophan uptake by your brain. But when insulin metabolism is not working properly, up goes another "Do-Not-Enter" sign; tryptophan has no way of getting through, and serotonin production breaks down. Without serotonin, you experience *craving instead of curbing* – your desire to eat continues. And now you have a biological and scientific excuse for excessive consumption of ice cream (or chocolate cake; mine is pecan pie).

So carbohydrate cravings can represent a deficiency of serotonin rather than a need for food.[35] And the tryptophan embargo and serotonin inadequacy continue. Impaired serotonin metabolism is at the end of a chain of events initiated by insulin resistance. A vicious cycle is under way. (*There's a hole in the bucket, Dear Liza, Dear Liza . . .*)

CALCIUM AND MAGNESIUM TO THE RESCUE

Calcium and magnesium are central to the solution of this syndrome because they work with insulin to regulate the flow of nutrients into your cells. According to new research, calcium may play a substantial contributing role not only in reducing the incidence of obesity, but also in minimizing the prevalence of the insulin-resistance syndrome.[36]

Magnesium also throws its weight around: This mineral plays a pivotal part in the secretion and function of insulin. One of the major reasons cells don't respond to insulin is a lack of magnesium. The higher the levels of magnesium in your body, the greater the sensitivity of the cells to insulin and the possibility of reversing the problem.[37]

Carolyn Dean, MD, in her marvelous book, *The Miracle of Magnesium*, points out that sugar overload can cause magnesium deficiency in several ways.[38]

Therefore, more problems: High levels of glucose can become toxic by causing the production of free radicals, which are electrically charged molecular fragments that can damage cells. To deal with these problems, your body stimulates your pancreas to produce even *greater* quantities of insulin.[39]

And even modest weight reductions, in the range of 5 to 10 percent of your body weight, can lower insulin resistance.

~~~~~

We need to remember our long evolutionary heritage. Wild foods – plant or animal – have naturally low amounts of calories and high nutrient density that serve as a natural check to obesity.

Health educators have a tough time persuading people to eat sprouted grasses or broccoli when chocolate, pop tarts, and sticky buns are everywhere. **We are already the fattest industrialized nation in the world.** If the present rate of increase in obesity continues, it has been predicted that *all* Americans will be obese by 2230.[40] This will certainly decrease the quality and long life that might have been anticipated for all of us.

We have the information we need to successfully treat many of the causes of obesity. Isn't that encouraging?

Yet no matter what lifestyle changes are recommended, whether they are derived from past or present experiences of populations, or from endless past or present reliable research, they seem almost irrelevant because they have been and continue to be very largely obliterated by the scent of fresh-baked bread or the taste of ice cream.

Chapter Five

CALCIUM FOR TWO:
MATERNAL MINERAL NUTRITION

WHY DO *I* HAVE BABY FAT?

More than 73 percent of women at a weight clinic indicated that they had retained more that 20 pounds following each of their pregnancies. It has been surprisingly difficult to identify strong predictors for weight development after pregnancy, mainly because pregnancy and weight gain are intertwined in a complex pattern. Factors involved include a change in lifestyle, such as eating behavior, physical activity, smoking cessation, and the duration of breastfeeding.[1]

The average weight gain after birth ranges from about 2 pounds to almost 7 pounds, with some women retaining as much as 35 to 40 pounds. For most women pregnancy heralds the seemingly inevitable beginning of weight increases that just won't go away. But it doesn't have to be that way.

Researchers reporting in the *Annals of Behavioral Medicine* suggest that weight gain retained after pregnancy is less likely to occur when the pregnancy diet includes unprocessed, natural foods, along with calcium supplementation.[2]

If I had only known about the calcium component when I was pregnant in the late 40s and early 50s, chances are I would not have had to grapple with those extra few pounds throughout the decades, a source of frustration that finally ended for me with the *California Calcium Countdown* formula.

An extensive study is currently under way to confirm the beneficial effects of calcium supplementation during pregnancy. Dr Daniel Hatton, Associate Professor of Behavioral Neuroscience at Oregon Health & Science University School of Medicine, the principal investigator of the study, made a statement that I would like to see placed in every pregnancy test kit, and read by all moms-to-be early on. Hatton said:

> There are many positive aspects to increasing calcium consumption during pregnancy. It would be great if such a simple and safe intervention was able to help women contend with body weight issues as well as provide for the child's needs. For many women, excess weight gain during pregnancy and then the failure to lose the additional pounds during the postpartum period **marks the beginning of obesity**. During this time of rapid weight change, it would be a great benefit if calcium could help curtail excess weight gain and facilitate weight loss following pregnancy.

CALCIUM AND PREGNANCY

The *American Journal of Preventive Medicine* reported that supplemental calcium during pregnancy is more than a means to protect against excessive weight gain. A 1200-mg calcium supplement taken during the third trimester at bedtime can significantly reduce maternal bone resorption.[3] A few other important associations follow.

Alcohol

We know a great deal about the effects of alcohol on the fetus, but little is known about the consequences for the mother if she drinks during pregnancy. A recent study shows that alcohol can disrupt calcium homeostasis and is known to have deleterious effects on bone.[4]

Calcium homeostasis

Maternal calcium homeostasis adapts during pregnancy to provide for the needs of the growing fetal skeleton.[5] This is fine for baby, but may contribute to a significant decrease in Mom's blood calcium.[6] One consequence? Weight gain!

Premature/low-birth-weight babies

The relationship between the levels of calcium and the risk of a child of very low birth weight were examined. There is significant protective effect of calcium intake on this risk.[7] Evidence links low-birth-weight to a higher risk of cardio-vascular disease decades later.[8]

Breastfeeding

Regardless of the dietary calcium content, the maternal skeleton is slightly affected by pregnancy but *severely* affected by breastfeeding. However, the degree of such response appears to depend not only on dietary calcium content, but also on the dietary calcium/phosphorus ratio.[9]

Women who breastfeed often complain about putting on an additional ten pounds of weight during the breastfeeding process. Large amounts of calcium are transferred to the offspring by breast milk. This demand results in a negative calcium balance in lactating mothers.[10] Could this be a factor in the increased weight? (Those extra pounds related to breastfeeding are usually lost when breastfeeding ceases, and now we know why.)

Calcium supplementation is associated with a reduction in blood lead levels among lactating women with relatively high lead burden. Pregnancy and breastfeeding mobilize lead stored in bone, which may be a hazard for the fetus.[11]

OUR UNACCEPTABLE BIRTH STATISTICS

Studies indicate a strong association between reduced calcium intake and pre-eclampsia, a very serious and common problem among pregnant women in this country, and one of the major reasons we have such poor birth outcomes. (Pre-eclampsia is marked by high blood pressure; it affects as many as 1 in 10 first pregnancies in the US, and 1 in 7 worldwide. If the problem advances to eclampsia, it can mean death for the mother and/or baby.) As indicated a few years ago in the *British Medical Journal*, this leads to the hypothesis that **the incidence of pre-eclampsia can be reduced with calcium supplementation.**[12] A more recent study demonstrates that calcium supplementation during pregnancy has been shown to prevent high blood pressure and preterm labor (two symptoms of pre-eclampsia).[13]

Despite nature's calcium preference for fetal health, our own infants aren't doing all that well when compared to babies around the world. Among our national health objectives in the US for the year 2010 is the reduction of our infant mortality rate to less than 4.5 deaths per 1,000 live births.[14] Currently, it's a shameful 6.7. If you look at the chart on page 91, you will see that **it is safer to have a baby in more than two dozen other countries.**

"You will lose a tooth for every baby." This old saying is still making the rounds, and there's a grain of truth to it. Well, maybe not a whole tooth. But when there isn't enough calcium to go around, your body knows where to find a plentiful supply: *your bones*. Contrary to popular belief, the most readily mobilized calcium is found in portions of bone, rather than teeth. When calcium requirements increase during breastfeeding, the message is: **"Do not pass Go. Proceed directly to Mother's bones."** And so the scene is set for Mom's fragile bone status in later life, *and* her weight problems on top of that.

BABY COMES FIRST

Even under conditions of a mother's extremely low consumption of calcium, the calcium content of her milk does not change; it appears to be entirely independent of the quantity in her diet. So if it's not in Mom's food, the calcium is served up from her bones.[15] The point is that nature recognizes the critical importance of calcium for the fetus, even going so far as to place the mother in jeopardy.

During the third trimester of pregnancy, maternal calcium absorption increases and the fetus accumulates about two-thirds of the total bone mass it will have when born. In early infancy, human milk calcium is derived primarily from maternal bone stores, which incur substantial bone losses that are quickly replenished during and after weaning – provided Mom is in good health, getting enough calcium, and avoiding calcium antagonists.[16]

Regardless of nature's heroic attempts, eventually the child suffers too. While calcium supplementation during pregnancy increases the health of our children with far-reaching effects, those children whose mothers have not received enough calcium supplementation while pregnant have a higher risk of increased blood pressure, already apparent when the children reach age seven.[17] In addition, the higher protein content in infant formula may cause an increased obesity risk in kids (compared with breastfed babies).

What Mom feeds her baby is of paramount importance for baby's future overweight risk.[18]

The scene is set for Mom's fragile bone status in later life, and again, almost certainly *her weight problems as well*. The preferential calcium treatment for the fetus over the mother is one very significant reason why so many women emerge from their pregnancies with added weight – too often the beginning of a problem that lingers for the rest of their lives.

It may be shocking to see that the US, one of the wealthiest and most advanced countries in the world, comes in at a dismal 25th on this list. This should serve as a clarion call to our government leaders and those in the medical community that when it comes to the health and well-being of our society's future generations, we are missing the calcium boat.

Calcium supplements taken by a woman during pregnancy could have a lasting benefit for her child's blood pressure. The investigators say such calcium intake may help "program" fetal blood pressure, possibly with effects that persist into adulthood.[20]

CALCIUM: THE ULTIMATE REGULATOR

Just for the record, here's a quick lesson on the importance of calcium, aside from its weight-controlling action. I promise, there won't be a test after the lesson. But hopefully you'll have a new appreciation for this remarkable nutrient, and you will understand why nature gives first dibs to the developing fetus over Mom when it comes to calcium handouts.

In addition to being the most plentiful mineral, calcium is also the busiest. Calcium is on life-saving call, 24-7.

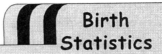

MEMOS

Birth Statistics

A SAD STATE OF AFFAIRS: OUR DISAPPOINTING BIRTH STATISTICS[19]

Country	Mortality per 1,000 births
Singapore	2.9
Japan	3.2
Iceland	3.4
Sweden	3.4
Finland	4.0
Belgium	4.2
Germany	4.5
Netherlands	4.5
Norway	4.5
Austria	4.7
Switzerland	4.7
Denmark	5.0
France	5.0
Spain	5.1
Canada	5.3
Italy	5.3
Luxembourg	5.4
United Kingdom	5.4
Australia	5.5
Ireland	5.8
New Zealand	5.8
Israel	5.9
Portugal	6.1
Greece	6.4
United States	6.7

From nervous-system communication and muscle contraction to regulating the flow of nutrients in and out of many cells, calcium is a critical factor in heart function, blood pressure, DNA synthesis and cell division, and, along with other minerals, it helps maintain acid/alkaline (pH) balance (explained in more detail in chapter eight.) It also plays an important role in blood clotting. It lines the walls of your cells. It controls the functions of very important enzymes. It is in charge of the production of certain essential proteins. Calcium even plays a key role in the detection of taste by the taste cells in the tongue.[21]

Supplemental calcium is often used to reduce heart irregularity and it can be helpful in treating congestive heart failure. It may decrease the risk of colon cancer. It may also protect against the dangers of mercury and cadmium – which are more prevalent exposures than most people realize. It does this by competing with these toxic minerals for cellular absorption sites.

As for your bones, Rudolph Ballantine, MD, another of our great pioneers in the field of medical nutrition, eloquently describes calcium's role:

> The skeleton of the body depends on calcium just as the more rigid, supporting structures in the earth's crust rely to a great extent on calcareous [calcium-like] formations such as limestone. The deposition of calcium in your bones is a structural process. It is almost as though your bones stretch up against the pull of gravity, raising us from the earth's surface. Without gravity, in fact, your bones begin to lose calcium. By the same token, when gravity is not exerting its effect and you are at rest, the calcification of the skeleton ceases, and calcium tends to be pulled out of your bones to be used for other purposes.[22]

If calcium intake is inadequate during growth, the full genetic program for skeletal mass cannot be realized. After growth, if calcium intake is inadequate, skeletal mass cannot be maintained. Because bone serves as our body's nutrient reserve for calcium, calcium is unique among nutrients: We walk on our calcium reserve![23]

Last but hardly least, as we now know, calcium helps to regulate the burning and storage of fat, and makes a major contribution to the feeling of satiety – the feeling of "having eaten enough."[24]

Although the recommendations for calcium have increased in recent years, we've still been suggesting a substantially lower calcium intake for ourselves than we feed our chimpanzees. Big mistake![25]

If you are an average healthy adult, you lose 500 milligrams of calcium from your bones every day. That's half a gram! At that rate, your bones would be reduced to powder in just a few years. What saves your skeleton is the fact that 500 milligrams of calcium are deposited *back* into your bone structure daily. Special bone cells called *osteoblasts* take calcium and phosphorus from your blood and deposit crystals into your bone structure. But other cells, *osteoclasts*, remove these same crystals and return calcium and phosphorus to your blood plasma. The outer layer of your bones – the calcium phosphate – is the material subject to the actions of these cells. This is very convenient; it makes the calcium readily accessible when needed.

Why this seemingly risky interchange of bone material *into* and *out of* your bones? Because it is extremely important for your body to preserve a specific concentration of calcium in your blood – a level that is maintained even at the expense of your bones. Nature considers the tasks for which calcium is responsible as matters of life and death, and so in nature's infinite wisdom, these tasks are given priority over your skeletal structure![26] This process also helps bone remodeling and repair by depositing calcium back to your bones.

YOUR INTERNAL UMPIRE

It's the last half of the ninth inning of the World Series. Your team is up, but it's down one run. There are three balls, two strikes, two out, and the bases are loaded. Here comes the pitch. Is it a ball or a strike? Will the batter swing or take the call? If he swings, will he hit it? Will it be a hit or an out? What about a close play at home plate? The outcome of the game depends on inches and seconds. One inch or one second can make all the difference.

And so it is with calcium in your blood! Just a small percentage either way makes all the difference. There may not be an office pool riding on your calcium balance, but your good health and even your life depend on this very precise, narrow range – so much so that your blood calcium cannot fluctuate by more than 3 percent![27] One inch and you win or lose the ball game. More than 3 percent, and it's your health, even your life.

Because calcium balance is a matter of life and death, you are provided with a very efficient internal umpire who calls the plays. Your everyday nutrition, however, can help or hinder the process. You need your best hitter at bat all the time to cover the crucial moments.

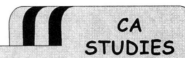

MEMOS

CA STUDIES

THE CASE FOR CALCIUM: STUDIES SUPPORTING CALCIUM FOR HEALTH

~ Calcium, vitamin C, and magnesium deficiency are associated with reduced bone mineral density in premenopausal women.
American Journal of Clinical Nutrition 2004[28]

~ Calcium may play a role in increasing levels of high-density lipoprotein (HDL cholesterol, the good kind), preventing colon polyp formation, reducing blood pressure in some hypertensive individuals, reducing kidney stone recurrence, promoting weight loss, and reducing the symptoms of premenstrual syndrome.
Urology in Nursing 2003[29]

~ The worst bone density status among women engaged in sports is found among dancers. Greater consumption of calcium could help this group avoid bone deterioration.
European Journal of Clinical Nutrition 2003[30]

~ Both animals and humans recover faster from infection with *E coli* (often responsible for traveler's diarrhea) when fed a calcium-rich diet, making them less likely to suffer from dehydration. It has previously been shown that dietary calcium (either from food or supplements) inhibits infection with salmonella.
Gastroenterology 2003[31]

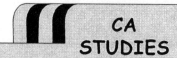

MEMOS

CA STUDIES

~ Low calcium intakes have been implicated over the last several years in a surprising variety of nonskeletal disorders.
American Journal of Clinical Nutrition[32]

~ The positive effect of total calcium intake on the bone mineral density of postmenopausal women suggests that supplemental calcium use is critical for maintaining bone mass.
Journal of Nutrition 2003[33]

~ There is an inverse association between high levels of calcium intake and colon cancer risk, meaning that the more calcium you ingest, the less your chance of developing colon cancer.
Cancer Causes & Controls 2000[34]

The National Academy of Sciences suggests that women aged 19–50 consume 1,000 mg of calcium per day and women over 50 consume 1200 mg per day.
American Dietetic Association 2003[35]

~ Calcium supplementation is a simple and effective treatment in premenstrual syndrome, resulting in a major reduction in overall luteal phase symptoms (the post-ovulatory phase).
American Journal of Obstetrics & Gynecology   1998[36]

MEMOS

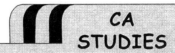

CA STUDIES

~ Calcium carbonate should be recommended as first-line therapy for women with mild-to-moderate PMS.
Canadian Family Physician 2002[37]

~ High blood pressure may be initiated in older women because of abnormal calcium metabolism.
Lancet 1999[38]

~ A high calcium intake will prevent calcium-deficiency bone loss.
American Journal of Medicine 1991[39]

~ Optimal calcium intake may increase bone mass and reduce the risk of osteoporosis.
Food and Nutrition Board, 1997
Report National Academy Press,
Washington, DC.

Calcium, Phosphorus, Mortar and Sand: Learning Ratios the Hard Way

Years ago, before my husband and I knew about the dangers of barbecuing, we decided to build a backyard barbecue. We bought bricks, mortar, and sand. We knew that the mortar and sand had to be in a 1:1 ratio to lay the bricks properly. We mixed the mortar and sand and added water to get the consistency needed. After spending a long day building the barbecue, we waited another day for the "curing" process.

To test the strength of the barbecue the next day, we pulled on a couple of corner bricks, and, much to our surprise, the bricks landed in our hands! At that point we decided to read the instructions on the bag of mortar. Uh, oh! It was a premixed product, ready for use. By adding sand, we had a ratio of 1:2, instead of 1:1.

This reminds me of the 1:1 phosphorus/calcium relationahip. Phosphorus, like calcium, is necessary for bone health, just as both mortar and sand are necessary for bricklaying. But if too much phosphorus is present, your bones, like our barbecue, will not have the integrity they need to keep your bones in good repair. Needless to say, we called a professional bricklayer the next day.

In the upper diagram on the next page you see a typical daily flow of calcium in and out of bone tissue. Less than a third of dietary calcium is absorbed.

In the lower diagram, you see a typical daily flow of phosphorus in and out of bone tissue. Absorption is above 90 percent, and excessive dietary phosphorus can interfere with proper utiilization.

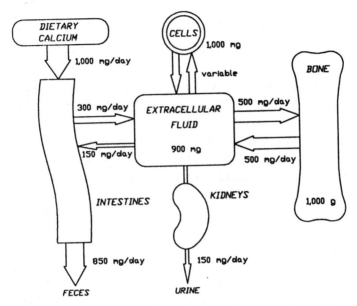

CALCIUM IN AND OUT OF BONES

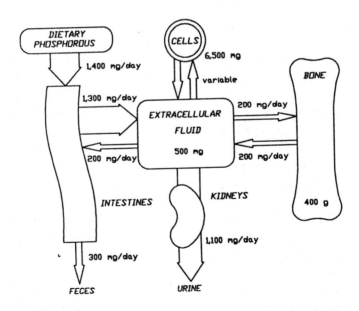

PHOSPHORUS IN AND OUT OF BONES

~~~~~

It has been shown that calcium supplementation during pregnancy serves to increase the health of children with far-reaching effects. Once again we see that calcium, along with its team of supporting nutrients, appears to be a key factor in both maintaining health and in managing proper weight. The two are inseparable.

Chapter Six

FAT FUTURE: BATTLING CHILDHOOD OBESITY

WHO EVER KNEW?

One day, years ago, I took my three young children to an ice skating rink after school. On the way home, I decided to stop for dinner at a new type of restaurant that had just opened – an inexpensive roast beef chain that welcomed children.

I will never forget the pleasure of that first-of-a-kind restaurant experience. The meal was no more costly than the dinner I would have prepared at home; my kids loved being able to make their own choices from a menu that included all of their favorite foods; and I reveled in the fact that I did not have to shop, cook, or do the dishes afterwards. I was certainly a more relaxed and pleasant mom that evening! In fact, our visit to this child-friendly eating establishment put us *all* in a good mood. All I heard on the drive home was, "When can we go back again?"

Little could I have predicted that almost fifty years later *on any given day* one out of three US children would be eating in what would come to be known as a "fast food" restaurant. As a result of my experience those many years ago, I have honestly always understood their appeal for busy parents. Unfortunately, this trend means our children are downing extra calories, sugar and fat at the more than 250,000 similar eateries that have covered the landscape nationwide.

Furthermore, the standards of the fast food industry have deteriorated over the years to today's low standards for taste and price, with little or no emphasis on nutrition.

Twenty-five years after our big night out, money spent on food away from home in the US represented 25 percent of the average family's food expenditure, while today it's more than 40 percent (with some estimates even higher). Needless to say, a huge amount of that is poured into fast food establishments.

US children who eat fast food today, compared with those who do not, consume more total calories, more calories per gram of food, more total and saturated fat, more total carbohydrate, more added sugars and more sugar-sweetened beverages at each meal – but less fiber, fruit and non-starchy vegetables.[1] Students in grades 9 through 12 (high school age) who eat at a fast food restaurant more than three times a week have calorie intakes around 40 percent higher than do those who do not eat at such outlets. That translates to a lot of extra pounds!

As the prevalence of overweight has increased in our children, so has their consumption of soft drinks. In adolescent boys, soda drinking more than *tripled* in the past three decades. Between 1977 and 1994, daily soft drink intake increased by 65 percent in adolescent girls and by 74 percent in adolescent boys. This is not surprising considering that the typical single-serving bottle of Coca Cola has increased in size from a fifth of a quart in the 1950s to two-thirds of a quart by the year 2000. There is also a trend toward guzzling more soft drinks as kids get older.[2]

Research validates the obvious: low physical activity and excessive television viewing are associated with overweight. In addition to significant changes in diet, the added combined effects of these two changes in traditional childhood behavior has also led to a large impact on unhealthful body weight.[3]

A survey of the eating habits of 3,000 youngsters aged 4 to 24 months found their diets to be surprisingly similar to that of older children – heavy on soft drinks, sweet candy, and other junk foods, and light on vegetables and fruits. French fried potatoes are the most common vegetable eaten by children 19 to 24 months old and 20–25 percent of these kids do not eat a single healthful vegetable; 25–30 percent eat no fruit. Soft drinks are being placed into the bottles of infants as young as seven months old, and most toddlers between 19 and 24 months consume sweets at least once a day.[4] They respond to the clang of the ice cream truck long before they can talk.

Obesity in *all* age groups is on the increase, and it's no surprise that US teenagers are the fattest in the world. *We lead the world in obesity figures of overweight children.*[5] Currently, one in six American children is obese.

It should come as no surprise that this rise in weight has been accompanied by the emergence of many serious health conditions. These include the classic cardiovascular risk factors: type 2 diabetes, menstrual abnormalities, sleep-disordered breathing, and psychosocial effects.[6] A Dow Jones newswire reported that 58.3 percent of children have one serious risk factor and 27.4 percent have at least two.[7] One in eight American children show *three* factors that point to a risk for heart disease.[8]

Heart attacks and other complications of cardiovascular disease do not usually strike until middle age or later, but these new findings add to growing evidence that the disease begins in childhood.[9]

Recent data demonstrate that nearly 30 percent of overweight adolescents meet the criteria for metabolic syndrome, described in chapter four. Approximately 910,000 US adolescents have metabolic syndrome.

NO DIETING FOR KIDS!

It is extremely important for a parent to understand why overweight children, unlike overweight adults, should not be treated with a weight-loss diet. Caloric restriction great enough to produce a weight loss will result in upsetting the metabolic balance that regulates a child's growth. (In adults, of course, growth is no longer a concern.) Studies have shown an inverse relationship between the rate of weight loss and the rate of gain in height over a period of six months or longer. Children on strict weight-loss diets grow less than their predicted rate, if at all. The needs of all essential nutrients increase with growth, and children who are severely restricted in their caloric intake fail to receive those adequate amounts of many nutirents.

Therefore, in treatment of overweight children, the goal should be *weight maintenance*, rather than *weight loss*. Eventually, as these children grow, their heights will reach appropriate levels for their weights and will equalize. They will literally "outgrow" the fat. (In some specific conditions, under proper nutritional supervision, an attempt to lose weight slowly may be made without jeopardizing growth.[10])

Children who frequently consume quality, whole-grain cereal (such as cooked oatmeal or millet) are less likely to be overweight. Cereal eaters have a lower body mass index and a higher nutrient intake than infrequent or non-cereal eaters. They consume more fiber and calcium and less fat than do those who choose other breakfast foods. For an average ten-year-old boy, the decision to eat good cereal or not can equate to about a 12-pound difference.[11] (This does not include the kind of "cereal" that can sit on a pantry shelf forever because no self-respecting bug would think of attacking it.)

Energy intake at breakfast affects performance on tests, memory recall and physical endurance in children up until lunch, as well as food craving throughout the whole day. This stresses the importance of a hearty breakfast for children and adolescents in the morning and a carbohydrate-rich snack at 10 AM to improve their attention, memory and willing participation in physical activities.[12]

High school girls with eating-disorder symptoms are much more inclined to smoke cigarettes, drink alcohol or use drugs than are those without such symptoms. Even middle-school girls (typically age 10 to 14) who have dieted in the previous month are almost twice as likely to become smokers as are non-dieters.[13] And eight-year-old girls with two obese parents are much more predisposed to become obese by age 10 than other girls their age.[14]

Blood pressure, insulin and cholesterol concentrations are higher in overweight children than in those with normal weight.[15] There is also an association with symptoms of wheeze and cough.[16] Being overweight is associated with an increased risk of new-onset asthma in allergenic boys and in nonallergic boys *and* girls.[17] The occurrence of allergy in children has many root causes, but childhood obesity is among one of the major risk factors.[18,19]

Additionally, weight problems in childhood most likely mean weight problems in adulthood – 80 percent of obesity in childhood and adolescence persists into adulthood, in spite of treatment.

Several studies point toward the role of soft drinks and fruit drinks in childhood weight gain in the US.[20] Based on what we now know about calcium antagonists, sugar overload, and allergies, the puzzle pieces should be starting to fit together. There is a solution – lifestyle changes in eating habits, exercise, and a boost from calcium supplementation can help resolve the problem.

TEEN AND LEAN

A nationwide study found that as many as one in four American children under the age of 14 is dieting. The same study found that children who diet gain *more*, not *less*, weight than non-dieters. This may be because of metabolic changes but more likely because they resort to binge eating.

So it's important for your child to know that dieting to control weight is not only ineffective, it may actually – and usually does – promote weight gain.[21]

Furthermore, those who are in the best cardiovascular shape as young adults are least likely to develop high blood pressure, diabetes and other cardiovascular risk factors later in life.[22] Teenagers who smoke but later quit have an increased risk of being overweight as adults. The strongest predictor of body mass index as an adult is body mass index as a teenager.[23]

Teenagers should also know about the association of obesity with breast cancer, skeletal maturation, exercise, menstruation, and calcium deficiency, all described below.

THE CALCIUM CONNECTION

Just as with adults, pregnant women, and the fetus, it's *calcium* to the rescue:

~ From the *Journal of the American Dietetic Association*:
A new study confirms the negative correlation between calcium and body fat. Research on more than 300 mixed ethnicity girls, aged 9 to 14, found that those who consume more calcium tend to weigh less and have lower body fat than those with low calcium consumption.[24]

~ From *Experimental Biology*:
Adolescent girls who eat more calcium weigh less and have less body fat than girls who consume the same amount of calories from other sources. The majority of American teens fall far short of daily calcium requirements.[25]

~ From the *American Journal of Clinical Nutrition*:
Small children may benefit from calcium intakes similar to those recommended for older children without adverse effects.[26]

~ From the *Journal of Bone Mineral Metabolism*:
Low calcium intake leads to decreased bone age and delayed pubertal development, indicating a link between calcium intake and skeletal maturation.[27]

~ From the *Journal of Adolescent Health*:
The consumption of sugar-sweetened beverages, sugars and sweets, and sweetened grains decrease the likelihood of meeting the Dietary Reference Intakes (DRI) for calcium. Only children who are nonconsumers of sugar-sweetened beverages have an average calcium intake that meets the adequate intake.[28]

~ From the *Journal of the American Dietetic Association*:
A varied diet is positively related to calcium intake, but intakes of carbonated beverages and other sweetened drinks are negatively related.[29]

~ From the *American Journal of Clinical Nutrition*:
Calcium supplementation for girls who have started their menstrual cycles and have low calcium intakes will enhance bone mineral integrity, especially in those who are more than two years past the start of menstruation.[30]

~ From the *Journal of Clinical Endocrinology Metabolism*:
The incidence of nutritional rickets appears to be increasing in North American infants and toddlers; it is widely assumed that

this is due to vitamin D deficiency. But low dietary calcium intake after weaning may result in the development of this disease, so attention to calcium intake as well as to vitamin D is essential.[31]

~ From the *Journal of the American Medical Association*: Forearm fractures are on the rise among both adolescent boys and girls, according to a Mayo Clinic study. It is theorized to be due to decreased bone acquisition caused by poor calcium intake.[32]

THE EXERCISE CONNECTION

The earliest sign of atherosclerosis involves a change in certain cells occurring in obese children as early as the first decade of life. However, exercise and resistance training can reverse this pathology, returning function to normal. But after eight weeks of inactivity, dysfunction begins to return as all of the positive effects revert back.[33]

Poorly-fit young adults are more likely to develop diabetes, high blood pressure and other ailments in middle age, placing them at greater risk for heart disease or stroke.[34] Exercise affects more than your child's waistline – kids who are less physically active and have excess body fat have more sick days.[35] Too bad the days of stick ball, stoop ball and hop scotch are over.

Obese adolescents are usually extremely inactive, which may explain why overweight teenagers can consume fewer calories than their normal-weight peers; they are eating more than is needed for their scanty muscular work.[36] Exercise and appropriate weight during adolescent years clearly delay the onset of breast cancer.[37]

Raise kids to play sports, and you may also raise future generations of healthier adults.[38]

WHY CHILDREN AVOID NEW FOODS

The refusal by children to eat new foods may not be due to fussiness but rather an evolutionary trait designed to protect them from harm. Babies will put almost anything in their mouths, but as children get older, they become more selective about what they eat, particularly if they have not tried it before. It makes sense that humans may have evolved to be highly suspicious of certain food types as youngsters. The problem is that strategies which were sensible for children to adopt thousands of years ago are not such a good idea now, and may be contributing to the low levels of vegetable and fruit consumption.[39]

SO WHAT'S A PARENT TO DO?

When dealing with children and food, the focus should be on changing the eating environment so that healthful choices become easy choices.

Instead of attempting to reduce calories, it is advisable to cut down on junk foods and to have large quantities of wholesome foods to make up for the deficit. The fruit bowl should always be full. A large bowl of assorted nuts (organic, and *in the shell*) should grace the kitchen table at all times. Oatmeal with cinnamon and bananas can become a breakfast favorite, and your overweight child should be told that he or she can eat as much of these foods as desired.

You might also consider getting your child to cooperate with you on the four-day elimination challenge described in chapter three. Make it a family affair – do it together. If your child proves to be sensitive to milk, cheese or peanuts (and the odds are high for that), it would be in his or her best health interest to eliminate these foods. Since you also don't want to encourage unhealthful dairy products, you might introduce quality probiotic yogurt. Served with fruit and/or nuts, it can be a nice treat. Nuts and seeds, sardines and other small fish, leafy greens, broccoli, whole grains, figs, salmon– all contain respectable amounts of calcium.

CALCIUM CONDENSED

Two large dried figs contain 80 milligrams of calcium, but it takes 156 saltine crackers to offer the same amount. One portion of raw green vegetables can have up to 250 milligrams of calcium. (Summer vegetables, by the way, have more calcium than fall or winter veggies.) Four ounces of salmon contain 291 milligrams of calcium, but it takes 73 cups of cornflakes (without milk) to fill you with the same 291 milligrams.

Children who eat with their families are more likely to consume fruit and vegetables, and to eat less saturated fat, fried food and soda.

In January 2004, officials in Philadelphia banned the sale of sodas throughout the public school system. Last year New York

City excluded soda, candy and sweet snacks from vending machines in its school system. California school districts are beginning to curb soda sales. If you live in a school district where soda flows freely, consider working with other parents to get these weight-inducing, calcium-depleting substances banished. For your child's sake, become an activist.

If you have kept an ongoing supply of soft drinks at home, there's nothing wrong with telling your children that you made a mistake, that you are now more knowledgeable, and that eliminating soda will not only make them feel better, but will give them more energy and help make their bones stronger. As a result, they have a better chance of doing better in their chosen sport.

Even if it's only fifteen minutes, try to take a brisk walk with your children as often as possible.

Again – it cannot be emphasized enough – be sure your children have a proper calcium supplement on a daily basis.

Explicit clear-cut limits are easier for children. Ambiguous restrictions are as confusing as no checkpoints at all. Children need boundaries that are in accordance with the values of the family. They want to know their parents care enough to set the parameters. The younger they are, the more captive your audience.

When children are young, they want to be like their mom and dad, rather than some actor or sports celebrity. Since children's role models change as they get older, the earlier you can alter your own eating habits, the better. That's when parental influence is greatest.[40] This of course, is easier said than done. But the suggestions offered later may help you to accomplish this goal.

CAUGHT BREAD-HANDED

For several Sundays in a row, the boxes of whole-wheat buns that we reserved for our weekend brunch had been pilfered. Sometimes one bun, sometimes two or three were missing.

It seemed obvious that the only culprit was our teenage son. (We were about to learn a lesson about the unreliability of circumstantial evidence.)

We talked to our son about his "hollow leg," and suggested other foods he could eat. We begged him to save the buns for our traditional Sunday feast, making it very clear that we did not appreciate the sneaky maneuvers he used to satisfy his insatiable appetite.

Our son steadfastly denied that he was the thief.

But one day the truth surfaced when we returned home earlier than usual, and caught our twelve-year-old neighbor in our kitchen, reaching into the freezer for the buns. (Our neighbors had our key on hand for safety purposes.) Jane was overweight, and her parents had placed her on a very stringent diet.

Coercion from parents can be counter-productive!

THE KITCHEN IN TRANSITION

While there is a growing awareness of nutrition, there is also a growing frustration in implementing food changes. Why the weak link between nutrition enlightenment and diet conversions? Because it's not easy! (One of my friends has said he would rather give up his spouse than his eating habits.)

Attempts at food changes may reveal the strength of the family. If you have a wholesome family structure with good relationships, the strain, if any, should be minimal. When parents have a high self-regard, children admire their parents and emulate them. Your children will have wonderful role models, and you won't have to sit down and tell them how to live. Everyone thinks it's cute to watch birds teach their young to fly. It's not only cute, it's vital. We teach best by example too!

Changeover is easy when children are young. A one-year-old doesn't make choices. As children grow older, *they* must learn to do the discriminating. They can only learn this through the education you provide. While the limits and goals you set are in transition, outlets and empathy are a necessity. The longer a food habit has been practiced, the more resistant to change that habit becomes. Allowing children to make choices – within the limits set – can help ease the frustrations of the food reforms.

WHO'S THE BOSS?

Children successfully get their parents to make purchases of *their* choice about 45 percent of the time. We can view this statistic as the optimist (the cup is half full) or the pessimist (the cup is half empty). Let's be positive: If 55 percent of parents can resist being manipulated by their children, *you can do it too!*

If you are making sudden changes when your child is fifteen, it is unlikely that your teenager will be entirely cooperative. You have probably thought about the changes for a while, and have come to the process of change through a process of thinking. Your decisions to alter food habits didn't *just happen* and it's really *your* journey. In your child's view, it's as though you were going along at 90 miles an hour, and suddenly slammed on the brakes – and there are no seat belts. Pow!

Meanwhile, the same time that you are saying, "Don't do it," the media and the culture are saying, "Do it. It's important. It's even sexy."

Of course, as a parent, you are in authority. You are in a position to set the limits. Your children do not have to agree with the curbs, but the burden of deciding on limitations is *yours*, not *theirs* (until they are older). Again, there's nothing wrong with saying, "No more." But you need to understand that your children will feel uncomfortable with your new ideas.

It is also essential for older children to be influenced by their peers. Children learn to develop a separate identity from you and your family largely through the influence of friends. You need to be able to treat your teenager's trip to the pizza parlor with friends as an important step in their social development, rather than an attempt to thwart your authority and values.

Although the struggles of teens with personal and social identity and peer influence may appear destructive (and sometimes it is destructive), it is a critical part of growing up. The more secure you are with yourself and your spouse, the more your children will assimilate your values.

But there is (and there needs to be) a limit to the control you have once your children leave the house.

Surprisingly, children come up with their own solutions that you may never have considered. One of my friends was being influenced by my family's eating habits. Her daughter was annoyed with her mom after being told she couldn't have soda and other junk food at her next sleepover party. The young lady sulked for a while, but then with the help of a friend and her mother, she came up with the fun idea of having an international pita party. The girls arranged a large basket of pita pouches surrounded by bowls of Mexican chili, Indian chicken curry, spicy Italian meatballs, Greek lamb chunks with raisins, and fresh salad.

The international theme gave the hostess clearance for serving healthful foods (high in calcium) with no apologies.

Keep in mind, too, that children feel victimized when faced with parents who do not present a united front. This, unfortunately, is a common problem. The best you can do is talk about the issue openly.

We must also acknowledge that our country has made very many mistakes in departing from natural nutrition. This is of prime importance for the evolution of the total acceptance of improved eating habits for coming generations.

MORE THINKING, LESS DRINKING

Cola increases in popularity with age. The fact that cola contains caffeine, an addictive drug, adds fuel to the flame: The more you drink, the more you crave. However, there is a decrease in cola consumption with education. Learning the effects of cola consumption has an impact on soda-drinking habits.

TEN SIMPLE TIPS TO LIVEN UP LUNCH

1. *Vary the food in the lunchbox*: No single food supplies all essential nutrients in needed amounts. The greater the variety in a single lunchbox, the less chance of nutritional deficiency. The diversity will also reduce the likelihood of exposure to excessive amounts of specific contaminants which might be found in any single food item. In addition, the repetition of foods and consumption of large quantities of the same food encourages allergy.

2. *Let kids do it themselves*: Wrap all the makings of a sandwich separately (use sectioned plastic containers with tight lids), and let children assemble the lunch themselves at school. For example, pack bread, dressing, sliced chicken, lettuce and cucumbers individually.

3. *Make food fun*: Festive foods should enter the lunchbox from time to time. One cute idea: animal cookie cutters on whole-grain bread to prepare nut-butter sandwiches in winsome shapes for younger kids.

4. *Go whole-istic*: Serve natural foods in their natural architecture. Pack a whole apple, a large chunk of bread (broken from an unsliced loaf), and green peas in their pods.

5. *Spice it up*: Spruce up bland mixtures using prepared mustard, fresh chives, horseradish, chili sauce, chopped olives, fresh oregano, etc.

6. *Go nuts at lunchtime*: Include nuts, seeds and legumes. Seeds are dormant plants, chock full of nutrients, waiting for the opportune time to grow. They are high in both protein and fat (the good-guy type of fat), and high in calcium. Include a nutcracker.

7. *Slice and dice*: Presentation often counts, especially with kids. Slip raw vegetables cut into small, attractive bits into their lunchboxes. Carrots, peppers, zucchini, cucumbers, squash, celery, and sweet potato are irresistible when cut into noodle-sized strips.

8. *Serve up some TLC*: Good food served with love! What a combination! As part of the trimmings, insert little notes which read, "I love you." "You are special." "Have a happy day." "Your teacher is lucky. She can be with you all day." Include TLC in the lunchbox.

9. *Go green*: Don't lock yourself into sandwiches only. Expose your children to salads. Include a small plastic tub of healthful dressing that they can add themselves at lunchtime.

10. *Make it a team effort*: Work with your kids to come up with interesting and delicious lunch ideas. Look through recipe books together; make them a part of the process.

EASY IDEAS FOR HEALTHFUL FOODS

Nut butter mixtures:

1. ½ cup nut butter, 1 teaspoon each: lemon juice, unsweetened coconut, sunflower seeds, sesame seeds, 3 chopped dates (or figs), 2 tablespoons shredded apple.

2. Add any of the following to the nut butter: grated raw carrot, alfalfa sprouts, peach and/or banana slices, sliced apples and/or sliced grapes

To prevent roof-of-mouth sticking, add a few drops of orange juice to nut butter mixtures. And, if possible, use organic nut butters free of hydrogenated or partially hydrogenated oils (a common ingredient in many name-brand peanut butters). Try almond, cashew, sesame and sunflower butters. Combine nut butters. Keep in mind that peanut butter is highly allergenic.

Fill whole wheat pita pouches with:
> Salad greens and grated carrots
> Yogurt with bits of raw broccoli and sprouts
> Shredded carrot, egg and avocado slices
> Homemade granola mixed with yogurt
> Grated carrots, eggs and chopped pecans
> Mashed baked beans with onion and small amount of grated cheese
> Greens, pineapple and nuts
> Salmon with chopped cucumbers
> Chicken and apple slices

Roll these fillings in a cabbage leaf instead of bread, or stuff into a green or red pepper.

Steam eggs to hardness by placing in steamer basket over boiling water. Turn heat down, cover pot, and experiment with time (every setup varies). An inexpensive egg puncher will pierce a pin-sized hole in the eggs, releasing air, thereby preventing eggs from cracking while cooking. Dye hard-cooked eggs to lend an air of festivity. Beet juice will dye eggs a nice bright red.

Dip grapes and banana slices in coconut, and then freeze. To keep frozen in the lunch box, pack with a small can of well-wrapped chemical ice (freezer gel in cans; available in hardware stores).

Scoop out celery sticks, zucchini, squash, cucumber, green peppers. Fill with nut butters, bean paste, grated carrot with raisins. Top with shredded raw cheese, caraway seeds, or sesame seeds. Place two halves together to close contents.

Add any of the following to plain yogurt: carob, unsweetened grape juice, vanilla, granola, nuts and seeds, vegetable bits.

For cold days, cut up fresh vegetables and place in a thermos with hot water, herbs, and bouillon seasonings.

These sandwich spreads are delicious on sprouted grain breads:
    Mashed avocado with buckwheat or sunflower lettuce sprouts
    Equal amounts of ground sesame seeds and soft butter, with a
        handful of sprouted lentils.

Buy fresh coconuts, and make the process of opening them a family project. (We used to place the coconut in a bag, and let the children take turns tossing the bag out of our second story window onto the front porch to crack the shell.) Store in the refrigerater, and break off pieces daily for lunch.

Invest in an inexpensive food dehydrator (which costs about $40 or less.) Dehydrated zucchini chips are a great substitute for potato chips. Any six-year-old can be in charge of the dehydration process.

Teach your children to sprout wheatberries, sunflower seeds, lentils, green peas, and garbanzos. Children love to see things grow quickly. (See Appendix C for easy instructions.) Jars of these tasty sprouts should be a kitchen staple. Add to soups, salads, and sandwich spreads.

~~~~~

Just as every human being is an integral part of a whole, so nourishment is a *gestalt* – a totality, and only its completeness can create well-being. Processed foods are mushed, mashed, and mangled, chipped and chopped. When we attempt to reassemble bits and pieces, we lose that integrity, and with it some good health. Think about this when you serve your child his or her next meal.

Put your weight behind your child's obesity problem.

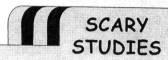

MEMOS

SCARY STUDIES

PARENTS: PLEASE READ

~ The pubertal growth spurt is associated with large increases in bone gain over a very narrow window of time. Approximately one fourth of the adult skeleton is accumulated in two years during the adolescent period. The potential of increases in bone gain with adequate calcium intake during this time is greater than at any other.[41]

~ Each additional soft drink a day gives a child a 62 percent greater chance of becoming obese.[42]

~ Pubertal adolescent females with vitamin D deficiency are at a significant risk of not reaching maximum peak bone mass.[43]

~ Total serum cholesterol level is negatively associated with height in pubertal children.[44]

~ Skipping breakfast appears to increase the risk of cavities in young children.[45]

~ Overweight children have significantly lower math and reading test scores compared with nonoverweight children in kindergarten.[46]

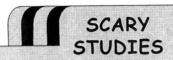

MEMOS

SCARY STUDIES

~ There is an association between a higher body mass index and symptoms of wheeze and cough in children, an association that appears to be stronger in girls than in boys.[47]

~ Dietary milk and its components, especially milk protein, have a much higher statistical association with hip fracture incidence than do other likely factors such as fat, protein, and sweeteners. What the statistical results show is that living in countries with a high dairy consumption is a risk factor for osteoporosis.[48]

~ The numbers of children with the hidden condition celiac disease, an intolerance to gluten, are significantly underestimated. The frequency of celiac disease at age 7 is the same as that in adults, suggesting that the condition starts in childhood, even in individuals in whom it is diagnosed late in life. We don't suddenly develop celiac disease – we've probably had it for years before it is eventually detected.[49]

Chapter Seven

THIS IS IT:
THE CALIFORNIA CALCIUM
COUNTDOWN FORMULA

THE FORMULA

Calcium. Magnesium. Potassium. Vitamin C. Vitamin K. Vitamin D3 (the hormonal form).

No matter what diet program you may have chosen, you should be able to shed those pounds more rapidly with the addition of a well-designed calcium weight-loss supplement. You may have to mix and match a variety of products to find all the important nutrients, but a good formula should have several of the ingredients listed above. A better formula will have *all* the ingredients listed above.

It is rare that anyone is deficient in a single isolated nutrient. It is just as rare for a nutrient to do its work all by itself. Studies of interactions among nutrients have been sparse, but just as variety in the foods you consume is paramount for optimum health, *a range of nutrients is essential for effective weight loss*. Focusing on one specific dietary component ignores the complexity of the weight-loss process. Your body needs all the help it can get! But that help must come from a combination of nutrients that make sense – an amalgam that is the result of scientific research and credible clinical experience.

MIGHTY MINERALS

CALCIUM

The use of calcium supplementation for weight loss has been described in previous chapters. Without magnesium and vitamin D, however, calcium can't function efficiently. Calcium, magnesium and vitamin D have been referred to as "the inseparable trio" for good reason: magnesium is necessary to convert dietary vitamin D into one of the hormones that makes efficient use of calcium.[1]

There is a link between stress and substance abuse, including food cravings. Since calcium is beneficial for lowering stress, it is understandable that it also plays a role in helping to reduce cravings and in promoting abstinence in those who want to be free of addiction.[2] Stress and physical exertion tend to deplete blood calcium, which leads to a vicious cycle of low blood calcium producing *more* stress, and *more* calcium depletion.

HEADACHE HELPER

Over the years, I have picked up many special "secrets" from highly reputable researchers with whom I have been privileged to interact.

Among my "gems": if you have an occasional headache or feel stressed, take six calcium/magnesium capsules, and take six more a half hour later. It has worked for me and many others every time! Calcium is a stress reliever, and the magnesium helps the absorption of the calcium.

Increasing calcium intake augments the amount of calcium absorbed, thereby protecting you from osteoporosis -- well, maybe. This effect depends on age, and it works best when you are younger.[3] To optimize absorption at *any* age, supplemental or dietary calcium should be spread throughout the day, with 500 mg or less being consumed at one time.[4] Imagine how much healthier Americans would be if *calcium breaks* replaced *coffee breaks*!

With an optimum calcium intake, you may reduce more than pounds. Increasing dietary calcium often results in reductions in blood pressure.[5] Recall, too, that insufficient calcium increases hormones that enhance fat storage.[6] See chapter five for additional benefits of calcium supplementation.

Caveat: beware of formulas that have *too much* calcium. Calcium intakes that are too high can increase the risk of serious disease states.[7] Depending on your age, the limit in supplemental form should be between 1,000 and 1,500 mgs. Dr Levine expands on this in the **Afterword**, on page 187.

CORAL CALCIUM

Primitive peoples found that they could relieve dyspepsia (stomach upset) by ingesting minerals with antacid properties. Calcium carbonate was among the first of these, as it occurred in relatively pure form in ocean coral.[8] Coral calcium is a natural mixture of many trace minerals deposited from the shells of sea animals. It is easily digested and there is a long history of testimonials endorsing its weight-loss attributes. The present data, although concluded from relatively few studies, suggest that the calcium that comes from coral is better absorbed than many other forms of calcium.[9] So the *California Calcium Countdown* formula includes coral calcium in addition to the tried-and-true form of calcium carbonate, the latter of which contains more elemental calcium than most other forms.

The research I did for my book, *The Remarkable Healing Power of Velvet Antler*, introduced me to the properties of glyco-aminoglycans (fortunately abbreviated as GAGs). GAGs are substances that include chondroitin sulfate and other good-for-your-well-being elements). I was fascinated to learn that coral adsorbs (attaches to, rather than absorbed into) GAGs because of its high calcium content.[10] GAGs help to lubricate joints in addition to playing other important regulatory roles.[11] Score two more points for coral calcium!

Ethnic Influences

With the same calcium intakes, African American girls retain more calcium than Caucasian girls through increased calcium absorption, decreased excretion and increased bone formation rates.[12]

MAGNESIUM

Calcium enters the cells by way of calcium channels that are jealously guarded by the mineral magnesium. Magnesium allows a certain amount of calcium to enter a cell to create the necessary electrical transmission, and then immediately helps to eject the calcium once the work is done. Why? If calcium accumulates in the cell, it causes toxicity and disrupts cellular function. Too much calcium entering cells can cause symptoms of heart disease (such as angina, high blood pressure and arrhythmias), asthma, or headaches.[13]

That's how Dr Carolyn Dean explains the role of magnesium in controlling calcium in her excellent book, *The Miracle of Magnesium*. Higher calcium and magnesium quantities allow cells to regulate and achieve optimal *lower* calcium levels within the cells. Calcium supplementation in the face of magnesium deficiency can lead to deposits of calcium in soft tissue such as joints. This promotes arthritis, or if the accumulation is in the kidneys, kidney stones. Too much calcium and insufficient magnesium can cause muscle twitches, spasms, and even convulsions. It can also tighten your bronchial tract (causing asthma), cause cramping in the uterus (leading to painful periods) and spasms in blood vessels (resulting in high blood pressure).[14]

KITCHEN SCIENCE

To understand how you can create a calcium/magnesium imbalance in your own body, try this experiment. Crush a calcium pill and see how much dissolves in 1 oz of water. Then crush a magnesium pill and slowly stir it into the calcium water. When you introduce the magnesium, the remaining calcium dissolves; it becomes more water-soluble. The same thing happens in your bloodstream, heart, brain, kidneys, and all the tissues in your body. If you don't have enough magnesium to help keep calcium dissolved, you may end up with calcium-excess muscle spasms, fibromyalgia, hardening of the arteries, and even dental cavities. And if there is too much calcium in the kidneys, and not enough magnesium to dissolve it, you can get kidney stones.

Reprinted with permission from *The Miracle of Magnesium*, Ballantine Books, 2003, C Dean, MD[15]

It has been proposed that premenstrual chocolate craving is widespread because magnesium is at its lowest around that time of a woman's cycle. Ounce for ounce, chocolate has more magnesium than any other food, and the irresistible urge to consume chocolate is presumed to be a sign of magnesium deficiency. The answer is not to eat more chocolate, but to increase magnesium intake. Dean indicates that chocolate cravings will vanish when there is enough magnesium in the diet.[16]

Since magnesium deficiency can compromise calcium metabolism and also hinder your body's production of vitamin D (further weakening bones), you can see the importance of magnesium supplementation for weight loss![17] Dean advises that "Current research seems to indicate that three parts of calcium to two parts of magnesium is probably most beneficial, with average optimal amounts of supplemental calcium at 1,000 mg per day and magnesium at 600 mg."[18]

A few more facts about magnesium, validated recently:

~ Magnesium deficiency is thought to be a risk factor for atherosclerosis,[19] whereas high magnesium (and potassium) intakes protect against this problem.[20]

~ Magnesium and potassium deficiencies usually coexist and also represent a risk factor for cardiac arrhythmias.[21]

~ Higher dietary magnesium intake may reduce the risk of developing type 2 diabetes.[22]

~ Magnesium keeps insulin under control; without magnesium, episodes of low blood sugar can result.[23]

~ Women with osteoporosis have lower-than-average levels of magnesium in their diets.[24]

~ Magnesium deficiency is associated with reduced anti-oxidants.[25]

~ Increased susceptibility to noise damage is linked to magnesium deficiency.[26] Low magnesium exacerbates noise-induced hearing loss, and increased magnesium intake provides a significant protective effect.[27] (Be sure you have enough magnesium before setting out for the Disco.)

POTASSIUM

> The greatest change in the human diet has been the increase in the dietary sodium/potassium ratio, reported as being changed by a factor of about 20.
>
> William Oliver, MD

Dr Oliver, emeritus chairperson of pediatrics, University of Michigan, is referring to the radical change in our diet, which has totally reversed potassium/sodium ratios to the detriment of our health and weight.

Potassium is found in abundance in uncooked fruits and vegetables – especially in rinds, husks, and stalks of edible plants, so its availability in natural foods is substantial. Sodium, on the other hand, is relatively scarce in natural foods. The hunter-gatherer ingested a diet high in potassium, but low in sodium. Perhaps that's the reason your kidneys easily remove excess potassium from your blood. Your metabolism is more frugal with sodium, simply because under natural conditions there is less of it to be found and eaten. Your body handles sodium with a more sparing kind of metabolism. *Your kidneys actually hoard sodium.*

As the numbers on the scale rise, it is likely that the sodium content of certain cells in your body have also risen. (It would be unusual that anyone who is overweight would be consuming foods high in potassium and low in sodium.) Those on quick weight-loss diets show a 20 percent reduction of the enzyme activity controlling potassium and sodium metabolism in their red blood cells.

On a calorie-deprivation diet, your body tends to decrease potassium levels and thereby blood sugar and insulin efficiency. So you are losing weight, but it's a catch-22 situation. When potassium supplementation accompanies a diet, however, better insulin and glucose utilization are the result. This is just one benefit for the potassium in the *California Countdown* formula,

Although weight loss is an important objective, *how* it is achieved is the critical factor.

Most people who are overweight often experience *fluid overload.* It's interesting to note that obesity is accompanied by an abnormal fluid ratio of potassium and sodium between the inside and outside of cells – something not observed in nonobese people. Proper functioning of sodium and potassium is important for weight maintenance because of its role in this inner/outer cell ratio.

ROLE REVERSAL: MODERN SODIUM/POTASSIUM RATIOS OUT OF WHACK

Following are but a few examples of how we have reversed the natural content of sodium and potassium in today's food.

~ Fresh corn has 289 milligrams of potassium and less than one milligram of sodium. Canned corn has 97 milligrams of potassium and 235 milligrams of sodium.

~ Potato chips have 250 times more sodium than the same amount of baked potato.

~ Dill pickles contain 238 times more sodium than a cucumber.

~ An average portion of fresh grapes has 158 milligrams of potassium. The same amount of reconstituted grape juice has only 34 milligrams of potassium.

This chart further demonstrates how the potassium and sodium content of natural and processed foods have been reversed:

POTASSIUM & SODIUM CONTENT OF INTACT & DISTURBED FOODS

In milligrams/100 grams food
(100 grams is approximately 3½ oz)

Food	Potassium	Sodium
Flour, whole	360	3
White bread	100	540
Pork, uncooked	270	65
Bacon, uncooked	250	1400
Beef, uncooked	280	55
Corned beef	140	950
Haddock, uncooked	300	120
Haddock, smoked	190	790
Cabbage, uncooked	390	7
Cabbage, boiled	130	230
Asparagus, raw	310	2
Asparagus, canned	250	200
Peas, fresh	380	1
Peas, frozen	135	115
Peas, canned	96	236

HOW POTASSIUM AFFECTS YOUR WEIGHT

A very important process that depends on the relationship of sodium and potassium is the regulation of calcium levels *inside* the cell. When there is a fairly high concentration of calcium outside the cell, and only a little bit in the interior, removing calcium from the cell requires moving it in an "uphill" direction.

The energy to accomplish this is supplied by what is known as the sodium/potassium pump. Without an ample supply of potassium in the blood between your cells, cell membranes can't generate the energy required to remove sodium from the cell's interior. The sodium will back up in the cell like cars on a freeway at rush hour.

The processes involved – meant initially for your survival in a very different dietary world of high potassium and low sodium – are no longer in your best health interest.

Again, surprisingly, a low amount of calcium in your blood does not have the effect of reducing the problem of high calcium in your cells. It seems that if calcium levels outside the cells are very low, the cells conserve calcium instead of pumping it out. It's analogous to behavior during a gasoline shortage. When gas is hard to get, you tend to get your gas tank filled whenever you can. Chances are you'll "top off" the tank every time you pass a gas station.

Anything that adversely affects your calcium metabolism adversely affects your weight.

A few more facts about potassium, validated recently

~ Potassium supplementation can reduce abnormal calcium excretion.

~ Potassium supplementation is known to increase urinary sodium excretion.[28]

~ Total body potassium is significantly related to total body calcium and bone density of the spine and radium.

~ A potassium-rich diet reduces blood pressure.[29]

~ A normal potassium diet can prevent many heart and kidney lesions, even though blood pressure remains hypertensive.

~ Caffeine causes an increase in urinary potassium excretion.

~ Athletes: a potassium dose has an effect on *future* exertions.

This section on potassium is excerpted from my book, *Everything You Wanted to Know About Potassium But Were Too Tired to Ask.*[30] If you are interested in learning more about potassium and how it affects fatigue, high blood pressure, the aging process, alcoholism and headaches, this book is a good resource. (More than one physician has told me they learned more about sodium and potassium and the sodium/potassium pump from this book than they did in medical school.)

STRESS AND MINERAL MAGIC

Dr. Hans Selye is known for his observations pertaining to stress. Among his numerous studies, he subjected test animals to severe stress, damaging their heart muscles. This caused the animals to die prematurely. But a control group under the same level of stress given magnesium and potassium had normal life-spans in spite of the stress.

VITAMINS OF VALUE

VITAMIN D

The roles of calcium and vitamin D are so intertwined that it makes sense that the requirements of either one of these nutrients depend on the adequacy of the other. Unfortunately, vitamin D deficiency is rampant in the US.

The major source of vitamin D is not diet, but sunlight exposure. (C'mon, ladies, get your bikinis on and get down to the beach.) Vitamin D is found in very few foods, most of which rarely find their way to the average kitchen table these days. (The list includes liver, cod liver oil or oily fish, egg yolks and butter.) Some researchers believe that total intake (from diet and the sun) should be 1,000 IU or even as much as 3,000 to 5,000 IU. (That translates to between 75 and 125 micrograms.) And if you are in good health and not a senior, you should be able to absorb this much through your skin.

In the aging population (65 years and older), and in particular for those who live in northern latitudes, vitamin D requirements are unlikely to be met sufficiently by sunlight exposure alone.

This occurs for two principle reasons:

(1) Skin pigmentation deteriorates with age, and so the conversion of the ultraviolet light on the skin is much less efficient.

(2) Older people do not spend as much time out of doors and are often covered up so that sunlight cannot penetrate the skin sufficiently.[31]

Recommendations to avoid all direct exposure to sunlight and use of sunscreen whenever outdoors are misguided and have serious health consequences. Adequate vitamin D could be achieved by exposing hands, face, arms and legs for about five to fifteen minutes daily between 11:00 am and 2:00 pm. Another way to restore sufficient vitamin D levels would be an oral dose of 50,000 IU of vitamin D once a week for eight weeks, followed by similar doses once or twice per month.[32]

FOR VITAMIN D, DON'T HEAD NORTH

Residents of Boston and the United Kingdom cannot synthesize vitamin D from November to the end of March. The half-life of the stored form of vitamin D is about three weeks, so Britons and Bostonians both become deficient by December.[33]

Vitamin D allows calcium to leave your intestine and enter your bloodstream. It works in your kidneys to help reabsorb calcium that otherwise would be excreted. When not taken in excessive doses, calcium and vitamin D have an excellent safety record.[34]

It was once thought that sunshine was a necessity to activate vitamin D, but new research shows that vitamin D supplements, *taken with calcium*, are sufficient.[35]

One of my favorite researchers on the subject of vitamin D and calcium, Hector DeLuca, PhD, points out that **the addition of a small amount of vitamin D3 causes a significant rise in calcium levels.**[36]

A few more facts about vitamin D, validated recently:

~ An unexpected risk factor for the potentially fatal falls suffered by older people has been discovered. *It's vitamin D deficiency.* Many women are so deficient that the same levels in a growing child would cause bone abnormalities. Supplemental vitamin D reduces the number of falls and the number of breaks caused by these falls.[37]

~ The evidence to support the role of adequate calcium and vitamin D for bones is strong. Maintaining blood calcium concentrations within the normal range is a priority and the major function associated with vitamin D.[38]

~ Oral administration of 1,25-dihydroxyvitamin D3 (the desired hormonal type) completely protects non-obese diabetic test animals from insulin-dependent diabetes.[39]

~ Combined with calcium supplementation, vitamin D appears to improve physical performance in older people.[40]

~ Vitamin D may prevent type 1 diabetes, and along with calcium reduce the risk of tooth loss.[41]

~ Vitamin D may reduce the risk of some cancers and provide an enhanced response to some chemotherapeutic agents.[42]

~ Calcium and vitamin D supplements seem to act synergistically to reduce fracture risk in both men and women; therefore, these supplements should be taken together.[43]

~ Vitamin D deficiency is common in patients with musculoskeletal pain.[44] Research has started to characterize the importance of vitamin D in neuromuscular function, especially among older adults.[45]

~ Calcium supplementation and vitamin D status appear to act largely together, not separately, to reduce the risk of colorectal cancer recurrence.[46]

~ Vitamin D may protect against rheumatoid arthritis.[47]

~ Vitamin D3 can modulate immune responsiveness and central nervous system function. It can act as a preventive agent against several malignancies including cancer of the colon.[48]

~ Vitamin D has been shown to kill prostate cancer cells.[49]

~ Vitamin D deficiency is the principle indicator in the debilitating disease, multiple sclerosis in women.[50]

VITAMIN C

If it had been up to me to name vitamins, I would have named this one first. It's hard to find any disorder for which no improvement is shown with the addition of vitamin C. This nutrient has an incredible number of different metabolic roles. So it's no surprise that it can also affect your weight.

Vitamin C is a water-soluble antioxidant, which means two things:
1. It protects complicated proteins from oxidation – that is, destruction that occurs by combining with oxygen.
2. It is easily carried to and from the places it's needed since it dissolves in water.

A report in the *American Journal of Epidemiology* showed that women who consume at least 500 mgs of vitamin C daily are at lower risk for breast cancer.[51] (Shouldn't this have been headline news?)

Among the lesser-known functions of vitamin C is its role in collagen, the flexible part of your composite bone structure. Vitamin C helps to repair collagen and to build it up. So an ample supply of vitamin C is important for good bone health.[52] Low intake of vitamin C has been associated with a faster rate of reduction of bone mineral density compared with women on higher doses.[53]

Vitamin C helps to assist calcium absorption, and can relieve allergenic symptoms.

About twenty years ago, Dr. Ewan Cameron, a physician and researcher who collaborated closely with Linus Pauling, attempted to duplicate experiments that had shown that vitamin C was useful against cancer. He and his associates discovered that five of their patients who had been on large doses of opiate painkillers (such as morphine) had a surprising result with the use of the vitamin C treatment. They now required only mild analgesics and not one experienced any withdrawal symptoms or made any requests that the opiate regimen be continued.

Linus Pauling, with whom I had an ongoing friendship and frequent "nutrition-dialogue" discussions, introduced me to Dr. Cameron. In addition to my personal interviews with Dr. Cameron, the story was publicized in a book by another innovative nutrition-oriented physician and good friend, Dr. Emanuel Cheraskin. Dr. Cheraskin also demonstrated vitamin C's capacity to control addictions.[54]

The importance of the buffered vitamin C in the *California Calcium Countdown* is clarified later.

A few more facts about vitamin C, validated recently:

~ Vitamin-C–supplemented test animals went through stages of fracture healing faster than a control group.[55]

~ Antioxidant supplements, such as vitamin C tablets, could become the new remedy for osteoporosis. Osteoporosis was recently classified by the World Health Organization as the second leading health care problem after cardiovascular disease.[56]

(Have you noticed that so many of the nutrients that help to keep our bones in good repair also help to keep our weight down? One study shows a negative predictor of body mass index with concentrations of vitamin C. That is, the more vitamin C, the less body mass index.[57])

~ Ascorbic acid (vitamin C) may be effective in reducing smoking and promoting smoking abstinence.[58]

~ Users of vitamin C supplements appear to be at lower risk for coronary heart disease, *but this is not true of vitamin C in the diet*.[59] (Sometimes reports in prestigious medical journals can be surprising. It isn't often you read that a nutrient is more effective in supplemental form than in food.)

~ Vitamin C inhibits the oxidation in HDL, preserving the antioxidant activity associated with this important good-fat component in your blood.[60]

~ High intakes of vitamin C have been associated with decreased incidence or severity of a number of diseases, including cancer and cardiovascular disease.[61]

~ Placebo-controlled trials have shown that vitamin C supplementation decreases the duration and severity of common cold infections, with even greater benefit for children.[62]

VITAMIN K

Vitamin K was discovered in Denmark and labeled vitamin K for the Danish word *Koagulation*. This vitamin does indeed help blood clotting and coagulation. It is found in nature and is made in the body. Consuming foods like yogurt and acidophilus or the Japanese fermented soy, *natto*, contribute to its internal production. (Freezing of foods, by the way, destroys just about *all* vitamin K.)

Whereas vitamin D stimulates intestinal calcium absorption, vitamin K supplementation stimulates kidney calcium reabsorption, helping to increase the integrity of your bones.[63]

A few more facts about vitamin K supplementation, validated recently:

~ Vitamin K1 supplementation retards bone *loss* in postmenopausal women between 50 and 60 years of age. If co-administered with minerals and vitamin D, vitamin K1 may substantially contribute to reducing postmenopausal bone loss at the site of the femoral neck.[64]

~ Low dietary vitamin K intake has also been associated with an increased risk of bone *fractures*.[65]

~ Vitamin K has been used to relieve pregnancy nausea.[66]

~ Children who get nosebleeds may be vitamin K-deficient.

OTHER NUTRIENTS THAT MAY BENEFIT A WEIGHT-LOSS FORMULA

CHROMIUM POLYNICOTINATE

Recently, advanced technology has helped us to discover a huge amount of new nutritional information. For example, enzyme activity can be examined within fat cells, recording changes as they take place in those who are overweight and also during weight loss (mind-boggling, when you think of the microscopic size of a cell). This previously unknown knowledge is quite useful. Recall the research showing that an enzyme in fat tissue sends a message to your brain to increase caloric intake as soon as weight loss takes place. Through recent advances in technology we now know that it's *too much insulin that initiates the communication between this enzyme and your brain.*

Insulin plays a major role in energy production. It affects weight control, helps to reduce appetite, curbs sugar and carbohydrate cravings, and enhances the body's capacity to burn calories. Overall, regulated insulin function increases the availability of glucose and decreases that of fat.

Without chromium, however, insulin's powerful fat-fighting properties may be for naught. **Chromium is essential for insulin performance.** Sadly, even our government agency, the Department of Agriculture, confirms that almost every American is chromium deficient. The main reasons for chromium's scarcity are excessive chromium losses caused by food processing, inadequate dietary supply, too much refined sugar and other simple carbohydrates in our diet, and/or your body's inability to convert chromium to its biologically active form.

In summary, chromium deprivation creates a chain of events involving impaired insulin metabolism that changes the way your body manages energy, thereby promoting weight gain. Chromium polynicotinate in supplemental form helps to resolve the problem.

OLIGOSACCHARIDES

Inulin and fructooligosaccharides (again, we are thankful for an abbreviation, in this case, FOS) are fiber-like substances extracted from the chicory root, which have been reported to stimulate calcium absorption. And you know by now that when more calcium is absorbed, bone resorption is suppressed, thereby improving bone mineralization.[67] FOS and inulin are referred to as *prebiotics*, which are non-digestible food ingredients that can stimulate the growth or activities of probiotic-like friendly bacteria normally present in the digestive tract and colon. This action is health-promoting. In addition to increasing the absorption of calcium, these particular prebiotics can also increase the absorption of magnesium.[68]

L-carnitine, beta-carotene, and glutathione are also among my favorite additional substances that can work either directly or indirectly in a weight-loss formula.

~~~~~

SO WHAT MAKES THIS FORMULA WORK?

On my radio show in New York City many years ago, I had the honor of interviewing Theron Randolph, another innovative MD specializing in environmental medicine. Dr Randolph explained to my listening audience that food sensitivities upset your body's acid/alkaline balance, thereby acidifying your system.

A buffered C compound (ascorbic acid with minerals), however, can often remedy this problem as it helps to correct that balance. Adequate doses can actually facilitate the elimination of an offending food. People often feel an immediate response of relief as the symptoms reduce or quickly disappear. Randolph was way ahead of his time.

The buffered vitamin C in the *California Calcium Countdown* formula is made so that when the minerals dissociate (come apart), the calcium, magnesium, and potassium ions (or molecules) are in the presence of an excess of ascorbic acid (vitamin C). (For the chemists among you, the minerals become CA^{++} MAG^{++} and K^+.)

This transforms the minerals in the supplement drink to *mineral ascorbates*, which we believe are better absorbed. They may also pass more easily across the brain, an extremely important fact because so many food reactions involve the central nervous system. Although the three minerals in their carbonate form are effective, their efficiency is compounded in the ascorbate form and with the alkaline pH (explained later). The combination of these elements – the minerals and the buffered vitamin C – produces something special and remarkable for symptomatic relief. It not only provides a quick fix, but it also balances the body chemistry (the pH).

You may have read about forms of calcium other than calcium carbonate being more absorbable. Calcium citrate produces more of an acid effect because of its strong citric acid component. Calcium phosphate not only adds an excess of phosphorus to your diet, but phosphate is an acid. These forms of calcium would interfere with the alkalizing effect of calcium, a key factor in the success of weight loss. Calcium carbonate is the superior form for our specific weight-loss goal.

Another pivotal point for the effectiveness of the *California Calcium Countdown* formula is the fact that the vitamin C is buffered. A buffering effect helps to neutralize excess acid. The minerals in the formula – calcium, magnesium and potassium – are alkaline. As explained, they counteract the acidosis caused by both allergenic and non-healthful foods.

You can see how the buffered C is a powerful tool for controlling food cravings by helping to keep your body's key minerals and its acid/alkaline pH in balance, the significance of which will be described in the following chapter.

Chapter Eight

SIZING UP YOUR FAT FITNESS

pH: A BALANCING ACT

ACID BLOOD?

Acidic blood may work for aliens, but here on Earth it can cause serious problems.

You've probably seen enough TV commercials to know that an "acid stomach" is not something you want to have. It turns out that a normal healthy body can utilize foods whether they are alkaline or acid because your blood acts as a "buffer" system to protect your normal pH.[1] But what does all that mean? Why should we know about it? And what does it have to do with weight loss?

In chemical parlance, pH stands for "potential" or "power." It comes from the German word *potenz*, and refers to the power of a solution to produce particular ions, or molecules. (See Appendix D for a more scientific explanation.) The important point is that acid/alkaline, or pH, is a term that refers to a condition in your body created by the food you eat.

Many abnormalities occur if the fluid outside your cells is too acidic or too alkaline. This concentration influences the speed of reactions in your body, how well your cells absorb nutrients, and even the structure of your cells.[2] So, yes, it is important to know about pH because it is a very significant indication of your health.

Foods that are processed (including candies and baked goods) plus meat, fats and a high-protein diet encourage acidity. People who have serious diseases are usually very acid. Rice, millet, vegetables and fruit help your pH stay more alkaline. (It's the *mineral* content of these foods that promotes alkalinity.) Vegetarian diets are significantly more alkaline than an omnivorous diet (a diet that includes meat), while a vegan diet (a strict vegetarian diet) is even more alkaline than a lacto-ovo-vegetarian diet (one that includes milk and milk products and eggs).[3]

Just as calcium in your blood must be maintained within a very narrow range, so it is with pH. Because your blood cannot (or should not) be too acid or too alkaline, you are provided with very tight controls. Your enzymes, immune system, and repair mechanisms do their best in an alkaline rather than an acidic environment, especially when it can maintain your pH at 7.4.

pH is measured on a scale of 0 to 14, with 0 being the most acidic and 14 the most alkaline. Again, when a solution is neither acid nor alkaline, it has a pH of 7, which is neutral. Pure water is chemically neutral, with a pH of 7. The pH scale is logarithmic, which means that each step is ten times the previous one. In other words, a pH of 5.5 is ten times more acidic than a pH of 6.5, and a hundred times more acidic than a pH of 7.5 (ten times ten).

When the pH of your blood is 7.4, the pH of spinal fluid is 7.4, and the pH of saliva is 7.4.

In the presence of too much acidity, guess what comes to the rescue? Calcium, once again. And where does it come from? *Your bones, if there isn't enough from ingested sources.* For the protection of the pH balance, calcium will leave your bones and enter your blood when needed. This represents a lifelong use of the buffering capacity of your bone.[4]

As already explained, resorption is associated very strongly with the loss of bone mass, which apparently nature deems as less important than maintaining a proper pH balance. The consequence of the bone resorption is considered a major contribution to the increased occurrence of osteoporosis. *Because meat and junk food assault your pH balance, you face a potential loss of bone integrity when you eat these foods.*

The extent of the bone loss caused by calcium defending your pH is not immediately noticed, but over a decade there could be a 15 percent reduction of inorganic bone mass in an average person.[5] For many years, folk medicine introduced people to the acid/alkaline bone concept: *clinical observation confirms that bone loss is greater under acidic conditions.*

But here's the good news: **A protein-rich diet is not deleterious to bone as long as it is accompanied by adequate calcium intake!** A calcium-to-protein ratio of 20:1 (mg of calcium to grams of protein) is recommended. This negates the need for calcium to be released from your bones

In addition to calcium, vegetables and fruits can act as buffers, or safeguards, to ensure that your pH balance stays within the normal range. These foods can reverse the urinary calcium loss that accompanies a high meat or high protein diet.[6] The potential acidity or alkalinity of foods refers to the *end* product after they are in your body.[7]

For example, Dr. Jarvis, Vermont folk medicine master, recommends apple cider vinegar for healthy bones. You may wonder why, since vinegar is acid. The alkaline reaction is caused by nutrients in the original apple, which contains all the micro- and macro-minerals that are responsible for triggering the alkaline response. (So an apple a day *does* keep the doctor away!)

The bicarbonate content of the *California Calcium Countdown* formula can help result in favorable changes in pH. Even the vitamin D in the formula helps to keep pH where it should be. Other buffers, or pH protectors, include brewer's yeast, lecithin, bee pollen, sprouted grains (mixed leafy greens), and kelp.

Urine of the herbivorous rabbit is alkaline, whereas that of the carnivorous dog is acid. Meat-eating humans usually excrete an acid urine while vegetarians excrete an alkaline urine.

WHAT ELSE AFFECTS YOUR pH?

Prolonged acidosis (an accumulation of acid in your body) may be present not only from continuous ingestion of large quantities of acid foods, but also from chronic kidney disease. And unless you're Peter Pan, there's the usual aging handicap: the ability of your body to excrete an acute acid load decreases substantially as you get older.

You can see why acid retention in seniors plays a role in the development of osteoporosis.[8]

Further immune responses – manifested as allergies, hyper-sensitivity and even stress – generate substantial amounts of acidic byproducts. Bone is continuously resorbed as a chronic response to recurring stress.[9]

Both where you live and your inherited tendencies also have their effects on your acid/alkalinity status. Even the very process of living produces a great deal of acid. When you eat you generate acid. When you move you produce acid. When you exercise you produce acid.

BUT WHY THE BIG DEAL WITH pH?

As indicated, proper alkaline balance is very important for bone health. We evolved in an alkaline ocean environment and even today our body's internal character remains alkaline. Blood must maintain a pH as close as possible to the ideal. At that level, cells are best able to absorb and utilize nutrients coursing through your body. The further the blood pH deviates from the ideal – that is, if it becomes too acidic or too alkaline – the less efficient many important metabolic processes become. The poor absorption of nutrients may begin to cause disorders like allergies, digestive problems or fatigue, and **weight gain**.[10]

All chemical processes have an ideal pH at which they operate most efficiently, and your body is no exception. For example, muscles operate best in a pH range of 6.9 to 7.2; if the pH is too acid – that is, lower than 6.9 – your muscles will feel weak. Your liver operates best at a slightly alkaline pH of 7.2 and your brain at 7.1. On the other hand, your stomach must maintain a highly acidic environment – a very low pH – in order to digest food properly (pH 1.5 to 3). If you're over fifty, there's a good chance you may have levels of stomach acid too low to completely digest your food. This means that key nutrients may not be digested and absorbed – and this includes calcium and the other nutrients needed for optimum calcium function. Low calcium levels can be a result of low stomach acidity.

pH BALANCE: FINDING NEW USES

Acid-base status is becoming increasingly important in nutritional medicine. Note the following:

~ A new toothpaste is being tested to fight cavities by promoting a higher pH in your mouth.[11]

~ In sports medicine, alkalization has been shown to increase the capacity for high-intensity exercise.[12]

~ The use of infant and preterm formulas that contain excessive amounts of acid equivalents was shown to cause growth retardation of infants.[13]

~ Similar negative effects can occur if inadequately composed synthetic amino acid mixtures and protein hydrolysates are consumed.[14]

~ Several kidney diseases require both control and manipulation of acid/alkaline status.[15]

~ Positive associations have been observed between rates of hip fracture and acid-producing diets.[16]

Because buffered C (as found in the *Calcium Countdown* formula) could decrease stomach acidity, it's a good idea to take buffered C between meals. It's important to use the buffered C when you feel unreasonable hunger, or when you experience food and chemical hypersensitivity reactions. But beware of overdosing; balance is the answer.

HOW TO TEST YOUR OWN pH BALANCE

Not unlike calcium or sodium/potassium metabolism, food-induced acidosis in those eating contemporary diets reflects a mismatch between the nutrient composition of the meal and genetically determined nutritional requirements for optimal acid/alkaline status.[17]

The typical American diet is usually too acidic because of our intake of animal foods, white flour, sugar, beverages such as coffee and soft drinks, drugs, and artificial chemical sweeteners.

Not only have the alkali-rich plant foods in our ancestral diet been replaced by cereal grains and nutrient-poor foods, but modern processing and food preparation have led to a considerable loss of nutrients such as potassium and magnesium, those wonderful alkaline minerals.[18] In fact, our current diet causes *lifelong, low-grade pathogenically significant systemic metabolic acidosis*![19]

And why should we care about this lifelong condition? Acidosis increases your risk for:

> cardiovascular damage
> kidney stones
> immune deficiency
> possible cancer mutations
> low energy
> chronic fatigue
> premature aging
> diabetes
> joint pain . . .
> weignt gain

Yes, an off-the-mark pH is another impediment to weight loss! (Why did you think we were talking about it to begin with?)

That's why there is an envelope attached to the inside of the back cover of this book. It has 15 pH paper strips so you can test your pH. Our medical community has yet to develop a foolproof method for measuring pH with precision accuracy, but these strips – sold in every drug store and used the world over – should give you a ball park indication of your pH level. It is not meant for diagnosis, but merely to give you a rather loose gauge so that you may compare your own results from time to time – especially before and after a diet change for the better (or worse). Instructions for use are on the last page of the book.

Caveat: If you are taking any drugs that influence your acid/alkaline status, the results may be distorted.

The best time to test your pH is about one hour before or two hours after a meal. It is recommended that you check your pH two days a week. The result of this saliva testing indicates the activity of digestive enzymes in your body, especially for the activity of your liver and stomach.

If you want to continue the testing after you use all these strips, you can purchase more at your local drugstore.

A half century ago we learned that *we are what we eat*. Then we began to realize that *we are what we assimilate*. The pH test may help you to see graphically that *we are also what our pH balance is*. If your pH is off the mark, you should give more thought to what you are eating and consider balancing your diet with the *California Calcium Countdown* strategy, especially if you are not absorbing nutrients properly from your diet.

Your diet can markedly affect your acid/alkaline status and your acid load can be specifically manipulated simply by dietary means.

FINDING YOUR BODY MASS INDEX

Old-fashioned ideal body weight tables have nowadays been replaced by the body mass index (BMI). Your BMI is based on your height and weight, and it gives a better – if still imperfect – body fat estimate. BMI applies to both adult men and women.

A person with a BMI between 25 and 29.9 is considered overweight, while someone with a BMI of 30 or more is obese. People with a BMI of 40 or more are classified as severely obese.[20] About nine million Americans have a BMI over 40![21]

To determine your BMI, divide your body weight in pounds by your height in inches, squared, and multiply the answer by 703. The following example is for a 5-foot 5-inch woman who weighs 180 pounds:

Step 1: Calculate the height in inches. (5 feet x 12) + 5 inches
       = 60 + 5 = 65 inches.
Step 2: Square the height in inches. 65 x 65 = 4225.
Step 3: Divide the weight in pounds by the height in inches
      squared. 180/4225 = .0426
Step 4: Multiply the answer in step 3 by 703.
      .0426 x 703 = 29.9

If you would like the math done for you, just log on to my webstie, www.bettykamen.com and click on the BMI button. This will link you to a program that does the calculation. Simply replace the sample data.

The seriousness of the complications of being overweight (that is, having a body mass index of more than 25) is an established fact. A new study published in the *American Journal of Clinical Nutrition* states that reducing BMI from more than 25 to less than 25 could eliminate 13 percent of America's obesity-related health problems, such as hypertension, diabetes, and hyperuricemia (excess uric acid in the blood, as in gout).[22]

BMI	WEIGHT STATUS
Below 18.5	Underweight
18.5-24.9	Normal
25.0-29.9	Overweight
30.0 and above	Obese

Between 1986 and 2000, the prevalence of a BMI of 40 or greater (about 100 lbs overweight) *quadrupled* from about 1 in 200 adult Americans to 1 in 50. The number of people with a BMI of 50 or greater increased by a factor of 5, from about 1 in 2,000 to 1 in 400. During the same period, the rate of moderate obesity roughly doubled, from 1 in 10 to 1 in 5. Obesity is no longer a rare medical condition. **A higher BMI in middle age is associated with a poorer quality of life in older age.**[23]

BYE BYE, HIGH BMI

Daily supplementation with the *California Calcium Countdown* formula is an effortless way to reduce your BMI. But you need a little more commitment and discipline to implement *The Working Strategy*, which is outlined in the next chapter. And, of course, there is exercise, which requires more push still. If you can commit to all three – the *Countdown Formula, the Strategy (which involves a few diet changes)*, and exercise, you will be doing something wonderful for both your weight *and* your overall health.

Physical activity has the potential to modulate your appetite control by improving the sensitivity of your physiological satiety signaling system (which translates to "more exercise equals fewer hunger pangs"). It can even alter your hedonic (pleasure-seeking) response to food.[24]

I have rarely met anyone who enjoys taking time out of their busy day to exercise. We can always think of something else we would rather be doing. As Carlton Fredericks, another long-ago nutrition guru, used to say: **"When I get the urge to exercise, I lie down until the feeling goes away."**

But a few new programs have burst on the scene and they are helping to change the negative attitudes many have towards working out. A favorite is *Curves*, the half-hour, three-times-a-week program for women. Programs like *Curves* recognize that it is counterproductive to give people goals they can't reach.

Sure, there is a dose-relationship between exercise and weight loss, but low amounts of moderate exercise, or about 30 minutes of walking per day, may be sufficient to prevent weight gain even in sedentary adults.[25] Walking aerobically (fast, but not so fast that you can't keep up a conversation) is also an excellent exercise endeavor. Daily walking is more likely to succeed if you arrange to walk with a friend.

By far, the most important finding that has emerged from exercise immunology studies is that positive immune changes take place during each bout of moderate physical activity. Over time, this translates to fewer days of sickness with the common cold and other upper respiratory tract infections. (These infections can increase when athletes push themselves beyond normal limits.[26])

A randomized trial published in the *Journal of the American Medical Association* advises that moderate exercise appears to be as good as vigorous exercise for reducing weight in sedentary women. Another study suggests that vigorous exercise may be no better than moderate intensity exercise in preventing breast cancer.[27]

When you supplement with the *Calcium Countdown* formula, your exercise program is off to a good start. Exercise generally causes a transient increase in circulating vitamin C in the hours following exertion, but a decline below pre-exercise levels in the days *after* the exercise. (These changes could be associated with increased exercise-induced oxidative stress.)[28] Dr Robert Cathcart, another one of the early alternative physicians so far ahead of his time, advises that we take vitamin C before exercising. The aerobic activity helps to get that vitamin C flowing through your body and into your cells.

MONITOR YOUR MEASUREMENT

Wearing a pedometer is a simple, noninvasive way to increase awareness of your daily activity and it has been shown to actually lead to increased physical activity. Maximum results in improved activity and better health occur in those who wear their pedometers *all the time.*[29]

The Surgeon General recommends that we walk 10,000 steps a day. An inexpensive pedometer lets you know in no uncertain terms whether or not you are meeting this goal. It gives you feedback all day long.

Using a small pocket tape measure to check your waist circumference is also a simple, inexpensive, and reliable way to check things out. Waist circumference is now accepted as a practical measure of adipose tissue distribution.

Your waist circumference should be measured by placing a tape measure around the smallest area below your rib cage and above your belly button.

Doctors are beginning to use such measurements in place of scale readings. By becoming a *waist watcher* you can compare your progress (or lack of it). The result is also an indication of whether or not you should be counted in the metabolic syndrome statistics.

Recall that abdominal obesity is one of the symptoms of Syndrome X. Increasing evidence shows that abdominal adiposity has a direct influence on health and that such fat correlates with health risks to a greater extent than does adipose tissue in other regions of your body. One report shows that waist circumference is more closely linked to cardiovascular disease risk factors than is BMI.[30]

WAIST NOT, WANT NOT:

<u>For Men:</u>
Ideal waist: between 31 and 36 inches
Overweight: between 36 and 40 inches
Obese: over 40 inches

<u>For Women:</u>
Ideal waist: between 28 and 33 inches
Overweight: between 33 and 37 inches
Obese: over 37 inches

Research shows that most people will underestimate the measurement when asked to share their number on the tape measure with someone else![31] No matter. As long as *you* know where you stand and what you have to do about it.

By age 18 the waist circumference in males larger than that of females, and this trend appears to continue throughout the years.[32] Recall in our discussion on Syndrome X that men should check in at around 38 inches; women at 45.[33] Research indicates the importance of using both BMI and waist circumference.

My very young grandson, watching us check out our BMI and our waist circumference, asked if this was the New Math.

~~~~~

The bathroom scale could now take a backseat when measuring your fat fitness. It is significantly less important than your pH, your BMI, or your waist measurement. These are more accurate ways for you to see just how well your body is working.

Chapter Nine

STRATEGY SIMPLIFIED

If you always do what you always did, you'll always get what you always got.
(Translation: Don't make any changes and you won't lose any weight.)

Don't expect to see the usual advice here, such as *increase your fiber* and *eat more whole grains*, or *consume five to seven portions of vegetables a day* or *be sure to eat those leafy greens* and *don't forget to exercise*.

Of course we should all be doing all of these things, but you would have to be a hermit or be living under a rock not to be bombarded with such guidelines almost daily. Not only do you already know about these recommendations, but you also know they are not so easy to put into action.

I promised you an effortless weight loss program. The first of my strategies may be all you require. However, the more of my ten suggestions you can apply, the better – for your *weight loss* and your *health*.

The proposals that follow are definitely more attainable. They won't force you to alter your lifestyle (not too much, anyway), but they certainly will have an impact on your scale readings!

#1. Add the well-designed *Calcium Countdown* formula to your supplement regimen.

Based on the extensive medical research presented here, this properly formulated and safe supplement can be taken once or twice a day – especially when *"I-wanna-eat-now"* or *"I wanna eat THAT now"* cravings surface and it's not even close to mealtime yet, but the refrigerator is beckoning.

Important Caveat: When you start a new supplement, always build up to recommended amounts gradually. If a supplement calls for a teaspoonful, start with a smaller quantity and give yourself time to work up to the suggested measurement. This is especially important if you have stomach sensitivity. Recall that the results of the Haight-Ashbury study demonstrated success in 90 percent of the participants with only 1½ teaspoons a day of a formula similar to the *Calcium Countdown*. A little goes a long way. On the other hand, if you are having a severe sensitivity or allergic response to something you ate or to something in your environment, a larger quantity has the potential to nip it in the bud! Use your intuition and common sense when it comes to quantity.

~Numero uno is the Calcium Countdown supplement.~

#2. Have a hearty breakfast.

Eating *early* in the day tends to reduce overall food intake, whereas consuming food *later* in the day increases input over the entire day. It may be that it takes more to make you feel full as the day progresses. So have a big breakfast. If you are among those who have absolutely no time for breakfast in the morning, check the quick breakfast idea in the recipe section. If you are not usually hungry in the morning, the trick is to eat less the evening before.

What is the reason for this phenomenon? The scientists theorize:
> Earlier in our evolutionary history, the [coming] of night greatly restricted activity. In modern times, however, the widespread use of artificial lighting has allowed people to remain active and eat late into the night. Could it be that obesity in the modern world results in part from the extension of the active period into the night when satiety mechanisms appear to be weak? If this is true, then a dietary regimen that encourages the ingestion of relatively large amounts of food in the morning and restricts intake during the evening might reduce overall intake and serve as a treatment or a preventative measure for those who are overweight.

Research shows that this is exactly what happens.[1] You can blame your obesity on the invention of the light bulb.

~ #2, eat a hearty breakfast.~

#3. Don't buy any fat-free dairy products.

This may fly in the face of common "wisdom," but remember that a small amount of fat is essential for calcium absorption, and the more calcium we absorb, the better our chances for weight loss.

Our country's fat-free craze has done nothing to help burgeoning waistlines anyway. Living cells and their working parts depend on *wholeness* to do their best job. You can't fool Mother Nature! Stop trying. When you do your marketing, think: *The less processed, the better. The more natural, the better.* Our metabolic pathways evolved while we were eating whole, natural foods. Fat-free is a far cry from natural.

~#3, stay away from fat-free dairy products.~

#4. Fermented dairy products, preferably organic, should be part of your diet every day.

Fermented dairy products are superior to their unfermented counterparts. Viable yogurt, kefir and buttermilk are preferable to the more commonplace milk and cheese. Liquid acidophilus (a tablespoon after every meal) or a probiotic yogurt such as Bio-K are among the best choices. Fermented food products increase the absorption of calcium, and you get a bonus of friendly bacteria.[2] Yogurt has more calcium than milk.

Dairy products exert a great effect on both fat loss and fat distribution.[3] But again, please select *fermented* dairy products. Probiotic yogurts are no longer a novelty product on supermarket shelves. According to the *American Journal of Clincial Nutrition,* lactose from unfermented dairy products such as milk and yogurt has the highest association with ischemic heart disease of any dietary macronutrient for men of all ages and postmenopausal women. Many commercial yogurts do not contain live bacteria by the time they reach your table. If you are confused about product brand, look for something like Bio-K, or check with a knowledgeable clerk at the health food store.

"And don't think that just eating more dairy can help you lose weight," advises Professor Novotny of the Department of Human Nutrition, University of Hawaii.[4] So don't overdo it!

This suggestion does NOT include cheeses, which are high on the allergy lists. An additional warning: high dairy product intake, in particular the high intake of cheese, is associated with an elevated risk of testicular cancer. Dairy products have also been linked to an increased risk of prostate cancer, and in women, breast cancer. The apparent increase in risk may stem from the high amounts of the female sex hormones estrogen and progestin (the synthetic form of the hormone) in our dairy products today.[5] When it comes to dairy (well, for any food for that matter), *organic* is the best investment.

The bioavailability of calcium from dairy sources is not considered to be greater than that of calcium supplied as nondairy foods, except for calcium from a few plant sources with a high phytate or high oxalate content, which, as described earlier, can interfere with calcium absorption.[6] (It may be that dairy products have some other attribute that affects weight loss – not yet identified.)

Because the enzyme lactase (required to digest lactose) is manufactured in the fermenting process, those who are lactose-intolerant are usually able to handle dairy products when they are fermented, as in viable yogurt (viable meaning that friendly bacteria are present).

> ~#4, avoid dairy products, unless they contain friendly bacteria, and restrict them to a small quantity consumed daily.~

#5. Switch from coffee to green tea – it helps to burn fat.

According to the *Journal of Nutritional Biochemistry*, green tea can speed up your metabolic rate, which helps your liver to function more efficiently. A recent US study of overweight men found that, with no other changes in their diet or exercise regimens, drinking green tea three times daily burned up 200 extra calories a day. Studies with test animals demonstrated the same results.[7]

> ~#5, switching from coffee to green tea is an easy call, unless you are absolutely forbidden to have any caffeine. (The caffeine content of green tea is far less than that in coffee.)~

#6. Include a small amount of "friendly fat" in your diet daily.

Believe it or not, friendly fat can help weight loss. In this regard, good choices include a quarter of an avocado, a handful of sunflower seeds, freshly ground flax seeds, or a tablespoon of grapeseed oil. Your brain is comprised of more fat than protein. (You can call me a "fathead" any time!)

Avocados, one of the most nutritious foods available, are an excellent source of raw fat, the kind most of us are deficient in. They are rich in monounsaturated fat, which is easily burned for energy. An avocado has more than twice the amount of potassium as a banana. Grapeseed oil has a mild flavor, a high smoke point, and lots of vitamin E plus other good nutrients. It is my choice for salad dressing and cooking oil, and is one of the most stable oils available.

Researchers are investigating how certain friendly fats – found in oily fish, beef, and lamb – may actually help to burn off fat that is stored in muscle and pancreatic cells, and therefore help to prevent metabolic syndrome in overweight people.[8]

> ~#6 advises the consumption of
> a small amount of friendly fats.~

#7. Keep a bowl of organic nuts in the shell on the kitchen table, especially almonds and walnuts.

Almonds are a good source of calcium. Walnuts are heart-protective. (They have an appreciable omega-3 content.) Studies indicate an inverse association between frequency of nut consumption and body mass index. Those on nut-rich diets excrete more fat in stools. In well-controlled nut-feeding trials, no changes in body weight are observed.[9]

> ~#7 is fun – keeping that bowl of nuts on hand will be enjoyed by your family and friends, too.~

#8. Prepare THE SOUP – often.

Want to get through the weekend or any holiday without piling on the pounds? Dig out the largest pot you have. Fill it halfway with water. Throw in an assortment of cut and sliced vegetables. Include any or all of the following: celery, carrots, sweet potato, squash, green pepper, red pepper, mushrooms, broccoli, spinach, zucchini, and peas. Add onions, 2 tablespoons tamari; dash pepper, oregano, thyme; garlic cloves (or crushed garlic).

Optional: Add a cup of wild rice, rice noodles, or basmati rice. Heat, but use a thermometer so that the water never gets above 118° F. (Enzymes are destroyed when temperature goes above 118°.) Let simmer on low heat for several hours.

Prepare THE SOUP on Saturday morning or at the start of a holiday and consume as much as you want throughout the weekend or during celebration days. (Be sure to put some of THE SOUP aside for Monday's lunch.) THE SOUP, plus the *California Calcium Countdown* formula, will put *you* in control of your food, rather than the *food* controlling you. If you use enough garlic, your house will be permeated with a delightful smell. Better cook extras for the neighbors.

> ~#8 advocates THE SOUP.~

#9. Learn to sprout seeds and beans, or buy organic sprouts at the health food store.

Sprouts provide the best way to consume food growing up to the minute of consumption. Sprouting increases calcium content. Sprouted lentils, for example, are very high in calcium.[10] See sprouting instructions in Appendix C.

A large bowl of sprouts costs only pennies. You may even be able to cut back on a few expensive supplements when you consume sprouts. Sprouted wheat berries offer the best possible vitamin E. (And, by the way, they're not fattening.) Alfalfa and chickpea sprouts may help eliminate the need for cholesterol-lowering drugs. The list of benefits goes on and on.

> #9 is worth the effort, even though it's not as easy to implement as most of the other strategies (unless you purchase ready-grown sprouts).

10. Eating grapefruit may impact the body's insulin levels, speeding up metabolism and leading to weight loss.

Eating a serving of grapefruit with each meal can lead to an average weight loss of 3.6 pounds if continued for twelve weeks, without other diet or exercise changes. Some lose more than ten pounds with the grapefruit-at-every-meal strategy. Grapefruit juice works, too, but it is not quite as effective. It is believed that the chemical properties of the fruit reduce insulin, which is known to help regulate fat metabolism. Since insulin plays a key role in diabetes, grapefruit may protect those who are overweight from developing type 2 diabetes.[11]

> #10, the grapefruit addition, has a long history of dieting success.

THE RECIPES

Most people have neither the time nor inclination to follow menu plans beyond a short period, even when they think a new plan will give them the figure they have been dreaming about. Those who do try to follow such plans are almost always back to their starting point in due course. Following the ten strategies may do more than any attempt at adhereing to specific menus. So there's no menu plan here, but I am sharing some special recipes.

These recipes are based on calcium absorption, good nutrition, fun, and good taste. Wherever possible, the ingredients used do not appear on the allergy list. Where eggs are included, try to purchase organic, fertile eggs from free-running chickens. Marshall Mandell, MD, a physician who also appeared on my New York radio show frequently, was another one of the pioneering environmentalists. He observed years ago that when his egg-allergic patients used organic eggs, they were free of symptoms that would surface had they used commercial eggs instead. His patients would call us while we were on the air to confirm their positive results when they followed Mandell's allergy or food sensitivity advice.

Rise and Shine

Let the *real* breakfast of champions step forward.

For the short-of-time breakfast noneaters, consider filling a thermos with hot water the night before, and add oatmeal (or any other whole grain), with a sprinkling of cinnamon. By morning, your cereal will be at the ready. Vary by slicing vegetables into the hot water in the thermos instead of cereal, and add a variety of seasonings. By morning, your lunch is ready to go work with you (and for you!).

any other whole grain), with a sprinkling of cinnamon. By morning, your cereal will be at the ready. Vary by slicing vegetables into the hot water in the thermos instead of cereal, and add a variety of seasonings. By morning, your lunch is ready to go work with you (and for you!).

Who says we have to have eggs for breakfast? Last night's leftover chicken or rice stir-fry are delicious, even cold.

GRANOLA

In the Beginning

4 cups rolled oats; 1 cup wheat germ; 1 teaspoon sea salt; 2 teaspoons cinnamon; 2 teaspoons nutmeg; 1 teaspoon allspice; ¾ cup vegetable oil; 1 cup honey; 1 teaspoon vanilla; 1 teaspoon almond extract; 1 cup chopped almonds.

In large bowl combine oats, wheat germ, salt, cinnamon, nutmeg and allspice. In separate bowl, combine oil, honey, vanilla, and almond extract. Combine both mixtures. add nuts. spread in large greased pan; bake at 350° for 20 minutes, stirring frequently. Cool and break into chunks. MAKES 6 CUPS.

Hint: Be sure to get your cinnamon at the health store. Most commercial brands of cinnamon are mixed with sugar.

On Your Way

Reduce wheat germ to ½ cup. Reduce salt to ½ teaspoon. Reduce oil and honey to ½ cup each. Add ½ cup sesame seeds.

Top of the Line

2½ cups rolled oats, 1½ tablespoons shredded coconut; 1½ tablespoons sunflower seeds; 3 tablespoons chopped almonds, ½ cup sesame seeds, 3 tablespoons raisins, drained, which have soaked in water several hours; 1 teaspoon cinnamon.

Spread grapeseed oil or vitamin E (break open a capsule) on baking pan. Combine oats, coconut, sunflower seeds, almonds, sesame seeds. Sprinkle on pan in shallow layer. Bake uncovered at 350° about 20 minutes, stirring occasionally. Remove from oven, add raisins and cinnamon. Cool and store in covered jar. MAKES 6 ½ CUPS.

BREAKFAST BAR
In the Beginning
6 eggs; 3 cups granola; 1 cup currants; raisins or dates (chopped); ½ cup almonds, chopped fine; ½ cup sesame seeds; ¼ cup sunflower seeds; 1 teaspoon cinnamon.

Beat eggs. Add remaining ingredients, mix well. batter will be thick. Let mixture sit 15 minutes while oven preheats to 350°. Pour mixture into well-oiled 9-inch-square pan. Press mixture into pan; smooth top. Bake 25 to 30 minutes or until lightly brown and firm. Remove from oven; cut into 1-by-2-inch bars while hot. Remove from pan by loosening edges gently with spatula. Cool. Store in airtight container. MAKES 3 DOZEN.

On Your Way
Reduce chopped fruit to ½ cup.

Top of the Line
Use "Top of Line" granola outlined above.

The Souper Bowl

A bowl of soup can be a hearty meal or a dieter's delight. Either way, a kettle simmering all day on "warm" provides a course or a snack at the ready any time of the day. (Caution: restaurant soup and canned soups are overdosed with salt.)

TARATOR SOUP
You and your guests will savor the best (and most healthful) soup you've ever tasted, giving you gourmet status.

In the Beginning
4 oz shelled walnuts; 5 peeled garlic cloves; 5 teaspoons grapeseed oil (preferably the garlic-flavored grapeseed oil); 5 cups plain yogurt; ½ cup cold water; 1 medium-sized cucumber, peeled and diced.

Mix walnuts and garlic. Add grapeseed oil, a few drops at a time, stirring constantly, until smooth. In bowl, beat yogurt

until smooth. Blend in walnut and garlic mixture and ½ cup cold water. Add cucumber. Chill inf ridge. Serve cold, sprinkled with finely chopped parsley or dill.
On Your Way
Sprinkle with finely chopped parsley or dill.
Top of the Line
Use only organic ingredients. SERVES 6.

LENTIL SOUP

Lentils have enough calcium to make them proud, and if they are sprouted, still more!
In the Beginning
1 16-ounce package lentils; 2 medium onions, slice; 2 medium carrots, sliced; 1 cup celery, sliced; 1 tablespoon sea salt; ½ teaspoon pepper; ½ teaspoon thyme leaves; 2 bay leaves; 8 cups water; 4 organic, nitrite-free chicken or turkey frankfurters (from the health store), cut in chunks.

1 ½ hours before serving, rinse lentils in running cold water. Discard any small rocks. In 5-quart saucepot over medium heat, cook lentils and all other ingredients except frankfurters. Again, don't let temperature go above 118°. Reduce heat to low. Cover. Simmer 1 hour or until lentils are tender. Discard bay leaves. Add frankfurters. Heat through. MAKES ABOUT 11 CUPS OR 6 SERVINGS.
On Your Way
Eliminate salt. Use only 2 frankfurters.
Top of the Line
Sprout lentils for 1 or 2 days before cooking. Save a few sprouted lentils to add to soup uncooked just before serving.

The Main Event

The best entrees do not appear in this section because they are so basic. For example, a meal of lightly steamed vegetables (steam only until the veggies reach prime color and are still crispy), and steamed fish or chicken, plus a large tossed salad containing 10 or 12 raw ingredients (including sprouts), embellished with whole fruit and nuts for dessert, is one of the easiest and most nutritious meals to prepare.

ORIENTAL RICE

In the Beginning

This dish has always been a favorite with my children. It's a meal-in-a-bowl kind of dinner, and it can be as varied as the seasonings in your cupboard.

1 tablespoon sesame oil; 1 cup rice; 2 cups water; 1 cup mushrooms; 3 tablespoons additional sesame oil; 1 cup chopped celery; 1 cup chopped green or red peppers; 3 tablespoons tamari; 1 cup diced water chestnuts; 1 cup green peas; 1 cup chopped scallions; 4 cloves mashed garlic; 2 cups bean sprouts; 2 eggs.

Place 1 tablespoon oil in skillet and heat. Add rice slowly, with heat still on, stirring continuously until each grain is coated with oil. (Note: this only takes a few minutes, but this unusual step will prevent grains from sticking together. Another method for avoiding grain-stickiness is to place 2 tablespoons of oil into the pot of water in which the rice will cook.) Pour water into another pot. Bring to boil. Add oil-coated rice slowly and cover. Reduce heat to lowest possible setting; cook 30 minutes. An old Chinese rice-cooking rule is: No peeking! (Lifting the cover allows steam to escape, and rice will not cook enough.)

Stir-fry mushrooms; set aside. Add remainder of oil and stir-fry celery and pepper (and any other vegetables such as broccoli or zucchini). Stir-fry only until vegetables reach prime color. Add tamari. Add rice and stir entire mixture. Now add water chestnuts, green peas, scallions, garlic, and sprouts. Lightly scramble 2 eggs and toss into mixture. Optional: add 1 or 2 cups of diced chicken or turkey.

On Your Way

Reduce tamari to 1½ teaspoons.

Top of the Line

Reduce tamari to ½ teaspoon. Do not sauté any of the vegetables. Add all vegetables in raw state after the rice is cooked.

DELICIOUS MILLET

Millet is a neglected grain in this country. One of my favorite breakfast dishes is a bowl of millet with sliced avocado. For something a bit more gourmet, here's "Delicious Millet."

In The Beginning

2 cups water; 1 cup whole millet; 1 cup chopped sweet onion; 3 tablespoons grapeseed oil; 1 chopped green pepper; 4 cloves minced garlic; 1 cup chopped mushrooms; 1 cup green peas and/or diced zucchini; 1 cup finely chopped carrots; ½ teaspoon salt; 3 tablespoons tamari.

Bring water to boil. Add millet; simmer, covered, on low heat, for about 20 minutes. In separate large skillet, lightly sauté onion. Add remaining ingredients, except tamari, Steam, covered, 5 minutes. Add tamari. Stir millet into vegetables. Heat through a few minutes more. Bake in 325° oven for 10 to 15 minutes or until top is lightly brown.

On Your Way

Eliminate salt and oil. Sprinkle millet and vegetables with sesame seeds and paprika.

Top of the Line

2 cups water; 1 cup whole millet; dash pepper; handful of sunflower seeds; 2 cloves minced garlic; sesame seeds.

Heat water to 118°. Add millet. Lower heat and cook, covered, 15 to 20 minutes or until all water is absorbed. Add dash of pepper, handful of sunflower seeds and garlic. Sprinkle with sesame seeds. Season with only as much tamari as necessary to reach acceptable palatability. Add raw diced vegetables.

LIVER SLIVERS

Liver is about the only organ meat we can get these days, but be sure it's organic. It's one of the few foods with a decent offering of vitamin D. (For those of you who are of my vintage and from the east coast, it was one of Carlton Frederick's favorites. He thought he didn't like liver until he tried this. Carlton Fredericks was a lone voice discussing nutrition a half century ago – the first mentor of many researchers like me.)

In The Beginning

½ pound organic liver; ½ onion, sliced thin; butter or grapeseed oil for pan; 1 apple, sliced thin.

Place liver in freezer 10 minutes to facilitate cutting process. Slice liver into thin, spaghetti-sized strands. Simmer onions in butter or oil. Add liver and apple slices. Stir-fry quickly, moving pieces about while cooking. Do not overcook. This is a fast process.

On Your Way

Garnish with sprouts.

Top Of The Line

Serve with lightly steamed vegetables for added nutrients and fiber.

The Side Dish

Don't sideline the side dishes. They may provide the missing link to add zest, fiber or nutrients to round out a meal. Side dish salads should accompany every meal, and if big and varied enough, could be the meal itself.

CARROT, CABBAGE, AND RAISIN SALAD

In the Beginning

1 cup finely shredded cabbage; 3 cups grated carrots; ½ cup raisins; ½ cup mayonnaise; ½ teaspoon sea salt; 1 teaspoon raw honey; 2 teaspoons lemon juice.

Mix vegetables and raisins. Mix mayonnaise, salt, honey and lemon juice. Stir all together well.

On Your Way

Eliminate salt and honey.

Top of the Line

Use only ¼ cup mayonnaise. Add sesame seeds.

MOCK CHOPPED LIVER

My mother used to make this a lot, and I was quite grown before I realized I was eating vegetables, and not liver pâté.

In the Beginning

1 pound fresh string beans; boiling water; 3 tablespoons grapeseed oil; 2 large onions, finely chopped; 1 stalk celery, chopped; ¼ cup walnuts, chopped; 3 hard-cooked eggs; 1 teaspoon chopped olives.

Cook string beans in boiling water until tender. Drain beans (save liquid for use in soup); set aside. Heat oil in skillet. Sauté onions until tender. Add celery. Cook 2 minutes longer. Chop beans, onion mixture, walnuts, and eggs. Add olives. SERVES 4.

On Your Way

Lightly steam string beans and celery instead of boiling.

Top of the Line

Use raw string beans and celery instead of cooked. Serve with other raw vegetables to upgrade fiber and nutrients.

Dressing It Up

Dress it but don't destroy it! Do-it-yourself embellishments enhance the flavor of salads without the need to post danger signs for stale and rancid oil. Here's a quick and easy salad dressing that takes five minutes: mash avocado and sunflower seeds and add a little grapeseed oil. That's it!

SUNFLOWER/YOGURT DRESSING

In the Beginning

1 cup sunflower seeds; 1 cup plain yogurt; 2 tablespoons chopped onions; 2 tablespoons chopped celery; 1 tablespoon dill.

Blend all ingredients.

On Your Way

Add chopped cucumbers.

Top of the Line

Add 1 tablespoon chopped alfalfa sprouts.

Fun Foods

For our dessert-oriented culture, we need good, healthful alternatives.

MINI-MARVELS

You will marvel at what these mini-marvels look and taste like. This recipe is especially helpful for the wheat-sensitive, and this recipe alone is worth the price of this book.

In the Beginning

3 eggs, well beaten; 1 cup chopped walnuts; 8 ounces chopped dates or raisins.

Mix everything together. Spoon into greased and floured *tiny* muffin tins. Bake at 350°, 20 minutes. Makes 24 small taste treats. Note: you must use mini-tins.

On Your Way
Soak raisins prior to use. Use fresh dates.
Top of the Line
Use freshly cracked, untreated organic walnuts, fertile, organic eggs, and organic raisins or dates.

PINEAPPLE YOGURT FREEZE

In The Beginning
1 cup plain yogurt; 1 cup crushed pineapple, unsweetened.

Place yogurt in freezer tray and freeze to mush. Remove. Add crushed pineapple and juice. Return to freezer. Freeze to soft mush. Place in mixing bowl; mix well. Return to tray. Freeze until solid. For variety, add strawberries, diced peaches, or unsweetened grape juice to yogurt. SERVES 4.

On Your Way
Use homemade yogurt or yogurt of superior quality.
Top Of The Line
Use fresh pineapple.

FRUIT CREAM DESSERT

In The Beginning
Chill or freeze any pieces of fresh fruit (bananas, berries, etc.). blend. Pour into ice cube trays. Freeze. Blend again. Freeze again. Top with yogurt, almonds, and coconut.

On Your Way
Use organic fruit.
Top of the Line
Use homemade yogurt, freshly hulled almonds, freshly grated coconut.

THE WEIGHT LOSS FRIENDLY FRIDGE

Crunchy Munchies

Carrots, celery sticks, red and green peppers, and jicama are low in calories and help keep cholesterol levels in check. The Iowa Women's Study found that the more carrots volunteers ate, the lower their odds of developing lung cancer, and those who eat carrots more than twice weekly may be half as likely to develop breast cancer as those who avoid carrots.[12]

High Calcium Foods

Keep the fridge stocked with good quality yogurt (Bio-K, for example), lots of bags of organic spinach, almonds, and broccoli. Other foods high in calcium include barley, crab, oysters, lamb, chicken, bok choy, kale, and beans.

Other Foods for a California Calcium Countdown Fridge

~ Vegetables and fruits help to reduce calcium excretion.

RESTAURANT CHOICES

Many diners report that bread dipped in olive oil is more filling than bread smothered in butter. A related finding was that nearly all of those queried in exit interviews underestimate how much bread they actually eat. This underestimation tendency is a consistent and well-documented phenomenon in consumption research.[13] In addition to eating more bread, the amount of oil used adds up to more calories than buttering the bread. (We always ask the waitperson to remove the bread basket when we are escorted to our table. It's easier to resist what isn't there.[14]

Questions to ask at *all* times, no matter what you are ordering:
1. Can you serve all sauces and dressings on the side?
2. Is anything I ordered fried?
3. Can I have doubles on the vegetables instead of the rice or pasta or potatoes?
4. Do you have fresh fruit for dessert?
5. Do you have bottled water?

Japanese women are regarded as the healthiest women in the world, averaging a lifespan at least five years longer than Western women. Frequent your local Japanese restaurant. (Older women may even find that their menopause symptoms will disappear if they go to a Japanese restaurant often enough, or use traditional Japanese foods at home.)[15]

And don't forget to take your *California Calcium Countdown* formula with you!

~~~~~

Good nutrition will give you a chance at a healthy old age. The weight loss offers a better chance at life itself.

AFTERWORD

Stephen A Levine

Calcium, the Satiety Messenger

A high calcium/alkaline diet and/or the use of the *Calcium Countdown* formulation provides satiety - a feeling of being full and satisfied. This finding fits the theories of the many experts who have demonstrated that higher calcium intake signals your metabolism to start burning fat for energy and heat. This calcium directive is letting your body know that it has enough food for necessary life functions, and that it can burn the surplus.

I believe this *satiety message* is a key signal that may even be referred to as the *missing link* to health and weight loss. The milk industry has certainly taken advantage of this generally understood finding with its "Got Milk?" series of commercials, telling us again and again that when we eat cake or cookies (or especially peanut butter), we've *gotta* have milk.

Not all things are good for all people. A small percentage may suffer from high alkalinity, or be exquisitely sensitive to *any* formula. And there's always the possibility of an ideosyncratic reaction. Different as we appear on the outside, internally we are even more varied.

Although the large majority do well with a formula like the *California Calcium Countdown*, follow Betty's advice to start slowly.

The one time "a little won't do ya," however, is for an uncontrollable craving.

References

Chapter 1

[1] Restack RM. *The Mind* (NY: Bantam Books, 1988), p 75.

[2] *International Journal of Obesity & Related Metabolic Disorders* 2003;10:1038.

[3] *Hypertension* 2003;42:474-480.

[4] *American Journal of Clinical Nutrition* 2003;78:928-934, 902.

[5] American Heart Association Scientific Sessions, Nov 2003.

[6] *Journal of Asthma* 2003;40(7):733-9.

[7] *Acta Med Austriaca* 1997;24(5):188-94.

[8] *Neuroimage* 2003;20(4):1964-70.

[9] *Journal of Nutrition* 2004;134:104-111.

[10] *American Journal of Clinical Nutrition* 1979;32:2723-33Supl.

[11] *Annual Review of Nutrition* 2003;23:147-170.

[12] *Textbook of Endocrinology*, ed Williams H (Philadelphia: WB Saunders, 1981), 907-21.

[13] *New England Journal of Medicine* 1974;291:178-85,226-32.

[14] Cheraskin E et al. *Psychodietetics* (NY: Stein/Day, 1974), p 36.

[15] *American Journal of Clinical Nutrition* 2003;78(5):928-934.

[16] *Sleep Medicine* 2003;4(1):21-7.

[17] *Archives of Internal Medicine*, Sep 22, 2003.

[18] *Journal of Clinical Oncology* 2004;22.

[19] *American Journal of Clinical Nutrition* 1989;49:937S.

[20] *British Medical Journal* 2003;327:1085.

[21] The Washington Post Co., 2003

[22] Novation Report, Hospital Purchasing Group, Dec 2003.

[23] *Monat Geburt* 1937;105:88-97.

[24] *Proceedings of the National Academy of Sciences*, USA, Sep 15, 2003.

[25] *Carbohydrates and Health*, Hood Lf and Wardrip EK, eds. (Westport, CT: AVI Publishing Co), pp 128-32.

[26] *Neuropsychobiology* 1987;17:19-23.

[27] *Neuroendocrinology* 1987;45:267-73.

[28] 16th European College of Neuropsychopharmacology Congress, Prague, Sep 22, 2003.

[29] *Endocrinology & Metabolism Clinics of North America* 2003;32(4):895-914.

[30] Doctoral study of Tanja Kral, presented at the North American Association for the Study of Obesity, Fort Lauderdale, FL, Oct 13, 2003.

[31] Rockefeller University Report, NY, July 5, 2003.

[32] *International Journal of Obesity*, Jul 2003.

[33] *British Medical Journal* 2003;327:700.

[34] *European Journal of Clinical Nutrition*, Oct 2003.

[35] *British Medical Journal* 2003;327:120.

[36] *Diabetes* 2003;52(11):2833-2839.

[37] National Health Interview Survey, *Health Affairs*, Jan 2004.

[38] *Journal of Medicine* 2002;33(1-4):247-64.

[39] *American Journal of Management Care* 2001;7(9):926-7.

[40] National Health Council Meeting, Dec 2003.

Chapter 2

[1] *Physiology & Behavior* 2002;79(3):347-52.

[2] *Ibid.*

[3] *Journal of Nutrition* 2003;133(1):249S-251S.

[4] *International Journal of Obesity & Related Metabolic Disorders*, Sep 16, 2003.

[5] *BioMed Central Cardiovascular Disorders* 2003;3(1):5.

[6] *Lipids* 2003 Feb; 38(2): 139-46.

[7] *Experimental Biology* 2000, Conference, San Diego, Apr 21, 2000.

[8] *Federation of American Societies for Experimental Biology* 2000; 14:1132-1138

[9] *Journal of the American College of Nutrition* 2001 Oct; 20(5 Suppl): 428S-435S; discussion 440S-442S.

[10] *Obesity Research* 2003 Mar; 11(3): 387-94

[11] *Journal of the American College of Nutrition* 2000;19:754-60.

[12] *Journal of the American College of Nutrition* 2002;21(2):152S-155S.

[13] *Journal of Nutrition.* 2003;133(1):243S-244S.

[14] I Garard, *The Story of Food* (Westport, CT: Avi Publishing Co, 1976), pp 166-67.

[15] *Journal of the American Dietetic Association* 2003;103(11):1513-9.

[16] *American Journal of Clinical Nutrition* 2000;72(3),758-761.

[17] *Osteoporosis: What It Is, How to Prevent It, How to Stop It*, B Kamen (NY: Pinnacle, 1984), p 34.

[18] B Kamen & S Kamen, *Kids Are What They Eat* (NY: Arco, 1983), pp 133.

[19] *Hormone Research* 2003;60 Suppl 3:71-6.

[20] *Journal of the American College of Nutrition* 2003;22(2):142-6.

[21] *Journal of the American College of Nutrition* 2003;22:201-207.

[22] *Journal of Physiology* 1998;511:212-322.

[23] Lecture presentation, B Kamen, Malaysia Palm Oil Symposium, 2002.

[24] 25th American Society for Bone and Mineral Research, Abstract SU259; Sep 21, 2003.

[25] *Journal of Clinical & Endocrinological Metabolism* 88:1043-1047.

[26] *Journal of Nutrition* 2001;131:2007-2013.

[27] Heiby WA, *The Reverse Effect* (Mediscience Publishers), pp 576-78.

[28] *Medical Journal of Australia* 2000;173 Suppl:S106-7.

[29] *Journal of Bone Mineral Metabolism* 2003;21(6):415-20.

[30] *Journal of Nutrition* 2001;131:1355S-1358

[31] Lijecnicki Vjesnik 2003;125(5-6):117-24.

[32] *American Journal of Clinical Nutrition* 1985;41:254.

[33] *Journal of Nutrition* 2003;133(1):2232-2238.

[34] *Journal of Nutrition* 2003;133(1):268S-270S.

[35] *Lipids* 2003;38(2):139-46.

[36] *Journal of Nutrition* 2003;133(1):249S-251S

[37] Experimental Biology Meeting, San Diego, Oct 2003.

[38] Ibid.

[39] Symposium, "Obesity: Weighing the Options, Toronto, Sep 2003, attended by leading scientists from the United States, Australia and Canada.

[40] *Medical Hypotheses* 2003;61(5-6):535-42.

[41] *Urologic Oncology* 2003;21(5):384-91.

[42] UT Southwestern Medical Center, Dallas, TX.

[43] *Journal of the American College of Nutrition* 2002;21(2):152S-155S.

[44] *Urology in Nursing* 2003;23(1):69-74.

[45] *Journal of Clinical Endocrinology & Metabolism* 2000;85(12):4635-8.

[46] US Government Code of Federal Regulations. Food and Drugs, 21. Part 101.54 (b). 1–4-2001. Washington, DC 2002.

Chapter 3

[1] *Journal of the American Dietetic Association* 1999;99(10):1249-56.

[2] *International Journal of Obesity* 1990; 14(9): 815-28.

[3] *Appetite* 1997;28(2):103-13.

[4] *Appetite* 1990;15(3):231-46.

[5] Baylor Medical College Report, Jul 2003.

[6] New Zealand Food Safety Authority Report, Jan 14, 2004.

[7] Rockefeller University Report, NY, Jul 5, 2003.

[8] *Obesity Research* 1995;3 Suppl 4:477S-480S.

[9] *Medical & Surgical Pediatrics* 2003; 25(2): 89-95.

[10] *Indian Journal of Medical* Science 2003 Feb; 57(2): 57-63.

[11] Personal interview with Theron Randolph, MD, pioneer of allergy research, WMCA, NY, 1980.

[12] E Cutler, *The Food Allergy Cure* (NY: Harmony Books, 2001), p. 15.

[13] *Otolaryngologic Clinics of North America* 2003;36(5):989.

[14] *Nutrition Reviews* 1984;42:216.

[15] *Lancet* 1989:493.

[16] Cochrane Database of Systemic Reviews 2003;4:CD003664.

[17] *The Physician & Sports Medicine* 1998;26(5).

[18] The Cleveland Clinic Department of Allergy and Immunology and the Department of Pulmonary and Critical Medicine.

[19] *Clinical* Ecology, ed LD Dickey (Springfield, IL: Charles C Thomas, 1976), p. 57.

[20] *Annals of Allergy & Asthma Immunology* 2003; 90(6 Suppl 3): 81-3.
[21] WebMD Scientific American® Medicine, Nov 11, 2003.
[22] *Annals of Internal Medicine*, 2003;139:802-809.
[23] P Philpott, *Brain Allergies* (New Canaan, CT: Keats, 1980) pp 24,25.
[24] University of Wisconsin Medical School Report, Jan 8, 2004.
[25] F Speer, *Food* Allergy (Littleton, Mass: PSG Publ Co, 1979), p. 2
[26] *Physiology of Behavior* 1992;51(2):371-9.
[27] *Acta Medica Austriaca* 1997;24(5):188-94.
[28] *Obesity Research* 1995;3 Suppl 4:477S-480S.
[29] *Appetite* 1998;31(1):9-19.
[30] *Appetite* 2003; 41(1): 7-13.
[31] *Journal of Nutrition* 2003;133(3):835S-837S.
[32] *Appetite* 1999;33(1):61-79.
[33] *International Journal of Eating Disorders* 2001; 29(2): 195-204.
[34] *Pharmacology, Biochemistry, & Behavior* 2000; 66(1): 3-14.
[35] *Journal of Allergy & Clinical Immunology* 2003;112:420-426.
[36] *Appetite* 1991;17(3):177-85.
[37] *Hormone Research* 1993;39 Suppl 3:72-6.
[38] *Appetite* 1997;28(2):103-13.
[39] *Addicitve Behavior* 1999; 24(3): 305-15.
[40] *Human Reproduction* 1997;12(6):1142-51.
[41] *Physiology of Behavior* 1999;67(3):417-20.
[42] *Appetite.* 1999; 32(2): 219-40.
[43] *British Journal of Clinical Psychology* 1995; 34 (Pt 1): 129-38.
[44] *Appetite* 2001;36(3):137-45.
[45] *Addicitve Behvaior* 1993;18(1): 67-80.
[46] *Australian & New Zealand Journal of Psychiatry* 1996; 30(5): 698.
[47] *Drug & Alcohol Dependendence* 1994;34(3): 225-9.
[48] Op cit, Speer.
[49] *Morbidity & Mortality Weekly Report* Jan 2004.

Chapter 4

[1] Price W, *Nutrition and Physical Degeneration* (NY: McGraw Hill, Sixth Edition, 2002).
[2] Price W, *Nutrition and Physical Degeneration*; (Santa Monica, CA: Price-Pottenger Nutrition Foundation, Inc., 1945), p 397.
[3] Ibid, p 401.
[4] Ibid.
[5] Ibid, p 402.
[6] Wilcox B et al, *Okinawa Program* (NY: Clarkson Potter, 2001). p 1.
[7] Kamen B, Kamen S. *Osteoporosis: What It Is, How to Prevent It, How to Stop It* (NY: Pinnacle), p 37.

[8] *Modern Nutrition in Health and Disease, 9th Edition*, 1999, eds CM Weaver et al., ed, Lippincott, Williams and Wilkins, p 141-154.

[9] *The FASEB Journal,* 2000; 14:1132-1138.

[10] *Journal of the American Medical Association*, Dec 18, 1994.

[11] *American Journal of Clinical Nutrition* 1991;54(1 Suppl):281S-287S.

[12] *Ibid.*

[13] *Journal of Clinical Endocrinology and Metabolism* 1996;81:1699.

[14] *Lancet* 1993;341:673.

[15] *Lancet* 1982;1:74-76.

[16] Kamen B, Kamen S. *Osteoporosis: What It Is, How to Prevent It, How to Stop It* (NY: Pinnacle), p 145.

[17] National Institutes of Health Report, Oct 10, 2003.

[18] AMA response to my book, *The Kamen Plan for Nutrition During Pregnancy* (NY: Appleton-Century-Crofts, 1981).

[19] Shils M et al., ed, *Modern Nutrition in Health and Disease*, 9th Ed. (Lippincott, Williams and Wilkins, 1999), Chapters 7,8,9,11.

[20] *American Journal of Clinical Nutrition* 2003;78:902-093.

[21] Bernstein R, *Dr. Bernstein's Diabetes Solution* (Boston: Little Brown, 1997).

[22] Reaven G et al.. *Syndrome X, The Silent Killer: The New Heart Disease Risk.* (City: Fireside, 2001).

[23] *Journal of the American Medical Association* 2002;287:356-359.

[24] Hebrew University Faculty of Medicine, Jerusalem, Jan 11, 2004.

[25] *American Journal of Clinical Nutrition* 1985;42:1063-71.

[26] *Metabolism* 1986;35:278-82.

[27] *New England Journal of Medicine* 1989;11:733-4.

[28] Challem J et al. *Syndrome X: The Complete Nutritional Program to Prevent and Reverse Insulin Resistance (City: John Wiley & Sons, 2000).*

[29] Kamen B. *The Chromium Connection* (Novato, CA: Nutrition Encounter, 1996), p 124.

[30] *American Journal of Physiology* 1969;216:1114-18.

[31] Guyton A, *Textbook of Medical Physiology* 5th ed (Phil, PA: WB Saunders Co, 1976), p 973.

[32] *American Journal of Clinical Nutrition* 1985;42:1063-71.

[33] *Neuropsychobiology* 1987;17:19-23.

[34] *New York Academy ofScience Annals* 1987;499:84-93.

[35] *American Journal of Clinical Nutrition* 1985;42:1240-45.

[36] *Journal of Nutrition* 2003;133(1):249S-251S.

[37] *Journal of Clinical Endocrinology Metabolism* 1998;83(12):4401.

[38] Dean C, *The Miracle of Magnesium* (NY: Ballantine Publishing Group, 2003), p 111.

[39] Challem J et al. *Syndrome X: The Complete Nutritional Program to Prevent and Reverse Insulin Resistance.* (NY: John Wiley & Sons, 2000).

[40] *Hospital Practice* 1997;32:123-48.

Chapter 5

[1] *Lakartidningen* 2003 Dec 4; 100(49): 4091-5. (Swedish)

[2] *Annals of Behavioral Medicine* 2003;6(2):149-159.

[3] *American Journal of Preventive Medicine* 2003;24(3):260-4.

[4] *Alcoholism, Clinical & Experimental Research* 2003;27(9):1507-19.

[5] *Annals of Clinical Biochemistry* 2003;40(Pt 5):508-13.

[6] *Archives of Gynecology & Obstetrics* 2003;268(4):309-16.

[7] *Environmental Research* 2002;89(3):189-94.

[8] *American Journal of Hypertension* 2003;16:801-805.

[9] *Calcified Tissue International,* Oct 2, 2003.

[10] *Journal of Clinical Investigation* 2003;112(9):1429-36.

[11] *Epidemiology* 2003;14(2):206-12.

[12] *British Medical Journal* 1997;315:281-285.

[13] *South African Medical Journal* 2003;93(3):224-8.

[14] *Morbidity & Mortality Weekly Report* 2003;52(36):862-6.

[15] Kamen B, *Total Nutrition for Breast-Feeding Mothers* (Boston: Little-Brown, 1986), pp 66-67.

[16] *Hormone Research* 2003;60 Suppl 3:71-6.

[17] *American Journal of Hypertension* 2003;16(10):801-5.

[18] Meeting of the Association for the Study of Obesity, London, UK, Nov 20, 2003.

[19] United Nations Population Revision 2002.

[20] *American Journal of Hypertension* 2003;16:801-805.

[21] *Proceedings of the National Academy of Sciences,* Dec 1, 2004.

[22] Ballantine R, *Diet and Nutrition* (Honesdale, Pa: Himalayan International Institute, 1978), p. 225.

[23] *American Journal of Clinical Nutrition* 2003;78(5): 912-919.

[24] *Modern Nutrition in Health and Disease,* 9th ed, 1999. Lippincott, Williams and Wilkins, pp 141-143.

[25] *American Journal of Clinical Nutrition* 2003;78(5): 912-919.

[26] Kamen B, *Hormone Replacement Therapy: Yes or No – How to Make an Informed Decision* (Novato, CA: Nutrition Encounter, 2002), p 80.

[27] Mervyn L., *Minerals and Your Health* (New Canaan, CT: Keats, 1980), pp 77-78.

[28] *American Journal of Clinical Nutrition* 2004;79(1):155-165.

[29] *Urology in Nursing* 2003;23(1):69-74.

[30] *European Journal of Clinical Nutrition* 2003;57 Suppl 1:S58-62.

[31] *Gastroenterology* 2003;125(2).

[32] *American Journal of Clinical Nutrition* 2003;78(5): 912-919.
[33] *Journal of Nutrition, Health, & Aging* 2003;7(5):296-9.
[34] *Cancer Causes & Controls* 2000;11(5):459-66.
[35] American Dietetic Association Report, Sep 17, 2003.
[36] *American Journal of Obstetrics & Gynecology* 1998;179(2):444-52.
[37] *Canadian Family Physician* 2002;48:1789-97.
[38] *Lancet* 1999;354:971-75.
[39] *American Journal of Medicine* 1991;5B:23S-28S.

Chapter 6

[1] *Pediatrics*, January 2004.
[2] *American Journal of Clinical Nutrition* 2003;78(6):1068-1073.
[3] *Archives of Pediatric & Adolescent Medicine* 2001;155:360–5.
[4] American Dietetic Association Conference, San Antonio, 2003.
[5] *Archives of Pediatrics & Adolescent Medicine.* 1/6/04.
[6] *Nutrition In clinical Care* 2003;6(1):4-12.
[7] Dow Jones Newswire Report, Orlando, Nov 11, 2003.
[8] Center for Research on Chronic Illness, University of North Carolina, Chapel Hill School of Nursing, Nov 9, 03.
[9] *Journal of the American Medical Association*, November 5, 2003.
[10] Personal interview with Dr. Fima Lifshitz, WMCA Radio, 1980.
[11] *Journal of the American Dietetic Association*, May 12, 2003.
[12] *European Journal of Clinical Nutrition* 2003;57(2):310-5.
[13] National Center on Addiction and Substance Abuse (CASA),Columbia University in New York. Dec 19, 2003.
[14] *American Journal of Clinical Nutrition*, December 2003.
[15] *American Journal of Clinical Nutrition* 2003;78(6):1068-1073.
[16] *Thorax* 2003;58:1031-1035.
[17] *American Journal of Epidemiology* 2003 Sep 1;158(5):406-15.
[18] *Annals of Allergy & Asthma Immunology* 2003 ;90(6 Suppl 3):53-8.
[19] Ibid.
[20] *Obesity Research*, November 2003.
[21] *Pediatrics* 2003;112:900-906.
[22] *Journal of the American Medical Association*, December 17, 2003.
[23] *Adolescent Medicine*, December 2003.
[24] *Journal of the American Dietetic Association*;103(12).
[25] Experimental Biology Meeting in San Diego, 2003.
[26] *American Journal of Clinical Nutrition* 1999;70(1):44-48.
[27] *Journal of Bone Mineral Metabolism* 2003;22(1):64-70.
[28] *Journal of Adolescent Health* 2004;34(1):56-63.
[29] *Journal of the American Dietetic Association* 2003;103(12):1626-31.
[30] *American Journal of Clinical Nutrition* 2003;78(5):993-8.
[31] *Journal of Clinical Endocrinology Metabolism* 2003;88(8):3539-45.

[32] *Journal of the American Medical Association* 2003;290(11):1479-1485.
[33] University of Western Australia, Perth, Nov 2003.
[34] *Journal of the American Medical Association* 2003;290:3092-3100.
[35] *Journal of Applied Physiology*, December 2003.
[36] *Nutrition Reviews* 1981;39:89-95.
[37] Women's Health Weekly, Nov 13, 3003, p. 2
[38] *Medicine and Science in Sports and Exercise*, December 2003.
[39] *Appetite*, October 2003
[40] ADAF Family Nutrition and Physical Activity Survey. Oct 2003.
[41] *Journal of Bone Mineral Research* 1999; 14:1672-1679.
[42] *Lancet* 2001;357(9255):505-508.
[43] *Osteoporosis International* 2002;13:S5.
[44] *International Journal of Epidemiology* 2003;32:1105-1110.
[45] *Journal of the American Dental Association*, January 2004.
[46] *Obesity Research* 2004;12:58-68.
[47] *Thorax* 2003;58:1031-1035.
[48] *American Journal of Clinical Nutrition* 1999;70(2):301A-302.
[49] *British Medical Journal* 2004;328:322-323.

Chapter 7

[1] *Journal of linical Endocrinolgy & Metabolism* 1985;61:833-940.
[2] *European Neuropsychopharmacology* 2003 Dec;13(6):435-41.
[3] *Journal of Clinical Endocrinology & Metabolism* 2000;85:4470-4475.
[4] *Clinical Geriatric Medicine.* 2003 May; 19(2): 321-35.
[5] *Journal of the American College of Nutrition* 2001; 20(5 Suppl): 428S-435S; discussion 440S-442S
[6] *FASEB Journal.* 14:1132-1138.
[7] Food and Nutrition Board 1997, National Academy Press, Washington, DC.
[8] *American Journal of Gastroenterology.* 1989; 84(2): 97-108.
[9] *Journal of Nutritional Science & Vitaminology*(Tokyo). 1999; 45(5): 509-17.
[10] *Biomaterials* 1999 Aug; 20(15): 1359-63.
[11] Kamen B, *The Remarkable Power of Velvet Antler* (Novato, CA: Nutrition Encounter, 2002), p 26.
[12] *Journal of Clinical Endocrinology & Metabolism* 2003;88:1043-1047.
[13] Dean C, *The Miracle of Magnesium* (NY: Ballantine books, 2003), p. 83.
[14] Dean, p 26.
[15] Dean, p 27
[16] Dean, p 127.
[17] Dean, p 140.
[18] Dean, p 231.

[19] *Stroke.* 2004 35(1): 22-7. Epub 2003 Dec 04.

[20] *Pathophysiology* 2003 Dec; 10(1): 1-6.

[21] *Fortschritte der Medizin. Originalien* 2002; 120(1): 11-5.

[22] *Journal of the American College of Nutrition* 2003;22(6):533-8.

[23] Dean, p. 6

[24] Dean, p 140

[25] *Indian Journal of Experimental Biology* 2002; 40(11): 1275-9.

[26] *Journal of the American Academy of Audiology* 2003; 14(4): 202-12.

[27] *Journal of Basic Clinical Physiology & Pharmacology* 2003; 14(2): 119.

[28] *Metabolism.* 2003; 52(12): 1597-600.

[29] *Journal of Nutrition* 2003; 133(12): 4118-23.

[30] Kamen B, *Everything You Always Wanted to Know About Potassium But Were Too Tired to Ask* (Novato, CA: Nutrition Encounter, 1992),

[31] 4th International Symposium on Nutritional Aspects of Osteoporosis; Lausanne, Switzerland, May 17-20, 2000.

[32] *Mayo Clinic Proceedings* 2003;78:1463-1470.

[33] *British Medical Journal* 2003;327:1228.

[34] *Urologic Oncology* 2003;21(5):384-91.

[35] Vieth R, *Nutritional Aspects of Osteopososis* (NY: Sspsringer Verlag, 2000), pp 173-195.

[36] F. DeLuca, Department of Biochemistry, University of Wisconsin, Madison, 10-22-03.

[37] NewScientist.com news service, December 2003.

[38] *FASEB Journal* 1988;2:224-236.

[39] Hector F. DeLuca, op cit.

[40] *Journal of the American Geriatric Society* 2003;51(9):1219-26.

[41] *Urologic Nursing* 2003;23(1):69-74.

[41] *Urologic Oncology* 2003 Sep-Oct;21(5):384-91.

[43] Ibid.

[44] *Mayo Clinic Proceedings* 2003:78:1463-1470.

[45] *Gerontology.* 2003 Sep-Oct;49(5):273-8.

[46] *Journal of the National Cancer Institute* 20033;95(23):1765-71.

[47] *Arthritis & Rheumatism* 2004;50:72-77.

[48] *Bioessays* 2004;26(1):21-8.

[49] *American Journal of Clinical Nutrition* 1999;70(2):301A-302.

[50] *Neurology,* Jan 13, 2004.

[51] *American Journal of Epidemiology* 1996;144:165.

[52] Kamen B, *Hormone Replacement therapy: Yes or No?* (Novato, CA: Nutrition Encounter, 2002), p 159-160.

[53] *Osteoporosis International* 2003;14(5): 418-28. Epub 2003 Apr 16.

[54] Cheraskin E, *The Vitamin Connection* (NY: Harper & Row, 1983) p167-8.

[55] *Archives of Orhtopedic & Trauma Surgery* 2001; 121(7): 426-8.

[56] *Journal of Clinical Investigation* 112:915-923 (2003).

[57] *European Journal of Clinical* Nutrition 2003; 57(2): 249-59.
[58] *Drug Alcohol Dependence* 1993; 33(3): 211-23.
[59] *Journal of the American College of Cardiology* 2003;42(2):246-252.
[60] *Journal of Nutrition* 2003;133:3047-3051.
[61] *Proceedings of the Nutrition Society* 2003; 62(2): 429-36.
[82] *Medical Hypotheses* 1999; 52(2): 171-8.
[63] *Bone* 2003;33(4):557-66.
[64] *Calciferous Tissue International* 2003;73(1):21-6.
[65] *Nature* (doi:10.1038/427493a).
[66] Wright J, *Dr Wright's Book of Nutritional* Therapy (Emmaus, PA: Rodale Press, 1985), p 415
[67] *Journal of Nutrition* 2004;134:399-402.
[68] Kamen B, *Everything I Know About Nutrition I Learned from Barley (*Novato, CA: Nutrition Encounter, 2003) p 140-142.

Chapter 8

[1] Albanese AA, *Current Topics in Nutrition and Disease, vol 3,* Nutrition for the Elderly (NY: Alan R Liss, 1980), pp 236-37.
[2] *Physiology*, p 888
[3] *Journal of the American Dietetic Association* 1985 Jul; 85(7): 841-5.
[4] *Lancet* 1968;1:958.
[5] *Lancet* 1968;1:958-959.
[6] *Review Therapeutique* 2000; 57(3): 152-60.
[7] Anderson L et al, *Nutrition in Health and Disease,* 17th ed (Philadelphia: JB Lippincott, 1982), p 65.
[8] *Journal of Laboratory and Clinical Medicine* 1968:72:278.
[9] *Journal of the American Geriatric Society* 1982;30:613
[10] *American Journal of Managed Care* 1997;3(1): 135-144).
[11] Association of Dental Research, Sweden 2003
[12] *European Journal of Applied Physiology & Occupational Physiology* 1999;80:64–9,333-6.
[13] *Acta Paediatrica* 1995;84:490–4.
[14] *Pediatric Research* 1977;11:1084-7.
[15] *Kidney International* 2000;58:1267–77.
[16] *The Journals of Gerontology. Series A, Biological Sciences and Medical Sciences* 2000;55:M585–92.
[17] *American Journal of Clinical Nutrition* 2002;76:16.
[18] *American Journal of Clinical Nutrition* 2003;78(4):802-803.
[19] *American Journal of Clinical Nutrition* 2002;76(6):1308-1316.
[29] *Annals of Internal Medicine,* December 2, 2003.
[21] The Washington Post Company, 2003.
[22] *American Journal of Clinical Nutrition* 2004;79(1):31-39.
[23] *Archive of Internal Medicine* 2003;163:2146-2148.

24 *Current Sports Medicine Reports* 2003;2(5):239-42.
25 *Archives of Internal Medicine* 2004;164:31-39.
26 Op cit, Current Sports.
27 *Journal of the American Medical Association* 2003;290:1323-1330, 1377-1379.
28 *International Journal of Sport Nutrition & Exercise Metabolism* 2003; 13(2): 125-51.
29 *Wisconsin Medical Journal* 2003;102(4):31-6.
30 *American Journal of Clinical Nutrition* 2002;76:743-9.
31 *British Journal of Nutrition* 1998;80(1):81-8.
32 *Journal of the American Medical Associaiton* 1990;263:2893-8.
33 *American Journal of Clinical Nutrition* 2002; 76(4):743.

Chapter 9

1 *Journal of Nutrition* 2004;134:104-111.
2 *Annals of Medicine* 1990;22(1):37-41.
3 *Journal of Nutition* 2003;133(1):252S-256S.
4 Experimental Biology Meeting, San Diego, 2003.
5 *International Journal of Cancer*, Oct 2003.
6 *American Journal of Clinical Nutrition* 2003;77(2):281.
7 *Journal of Nutritional Biochemistry* 2003;14(11):671-6.
8 Association for the Study of Obesity Meeting, London, Nov 20, 2003.
9 *American Journal of Clinical Nutrition* 2003;78(3):647S-650S.
10 *Journal of Nutrition* 2003;133:2728.
11 Scripps Clinic Nutrition & Metabolic Research Center Report, Jan 29, 2004.
12 *Epidemiology* 1998;9(3).
13 *International Journal of* Obesity, July 2003.
14 Ibid.
15 Australasian Menopause Conference, Hobart, Australia, Nov 2003.

Appendix A

HAIGHT-ASHBURY FREE MEDICAL CLINIC

EFFICACY OF BUFFERED ASCORBATE COMPOUND (BAC) IN THE DETOXIFICATION AND AFTERCARE OF CLIENTS INVOLVED IN OPIATE AND STIMULANT ABUSE

Former Director   John Newmeyer, PhD
Project Director   Darryl Inaba, PhD
Medical Director   David E Smith, MD
Research   Gary E Waldorf, PhD
     Stephen A Levine, PhD

Product Design Research Survey Developed & Funded by
Allergy Research Group

EXCERPTS FROM STUDY

This pilot study suggests that a significant benefit was obtained from the clients participating in the study when using BAC in their detoxification and aftercare programs. This benefit was seen in rapid relief of acute withdrawal symptoms as well as discouraging resumption of drug abuse.

In general, reduced withdrawal symptoms were reported by most clients with those in aftercare reporting a remarkable 90% loss of craving for the specific substance they were abusing. The longer the client used the BAC, the more benefit they derived from it. Those who missed taking the compound felt a significant letdown and resumed the use of the BAC. There was a very low dropout rate (less than 1%).

There are many advantages of the BAC for use in treatment of drug abusers. It is easily and economically administered, and patients need not be hospitalized during treatment. It can be carried with the client. Counseling is feasible throughout the treatment program as clients remain alert and physical health appears to be enhanced. No serious side effects have been noted.

Appendix B

The Weston A. Price Foundation for Wise Traditions in Food, Farming and the Healing Arts

From the Web site: "The Weston A. Price Foundation is a nonprofit, tax-exempt charity founded in 1999 to disseminate the research of nutrition pioneer Dr. Weston Price, whose studies of isolated non-industrialized peoples established the parameters of human health and determined the optimum characteristics of human diets.

"The Foundation is dedicated to restoring nutrient-dense foods to the human diet through education, research and activism. It supports a number of movements that contribute to this objective including accurate nutrition instruction, organic and biodynamic farming, pasture-feeding of livestock, community-supported farms, honest and informative labeling, prepared parenting and nurturing therapies."

The Price Foundation supports dairies that do not pasteurize their milk. At their website, you will find powerful arguments in favor of raw milk and raw milk products from certified, healthy cows. These articles target pasteurization as the cause of many health problems associated with milk.

Appendix C

SPROUTING

A seed or bean will start to *germinate* (sprout or grow) when exposed to the proper conditions of air, light, and humidity. By creating these conditions, you become an indoor farmer.

Simple Sprouting

- 1. Soak 1 or 2 tbsp of seeds or beans in 1 cup of water overnight.

- 2. In the morning, pour the water off (don't discard the water; feed it to your plants – they will love it!) and rinse the seeds under the faucet using luke warm water. The easiest procedure is to place the seeds in a strainer for rinsing.

- 3. Place the seeds in a glass jar. Cover the jar with nylon netting (available at any hardware or fabric store), and secure the netting with a rubber band.

- 4. Tilt the jar at an angle in your dish rack, so that any excess water will run off. Sprouts like moisture, but not puddles.

- 5. Rinse the seeds once or twice each day (three or four times if you are home and have the time). You may find it easier to dump the seeds into a strainer, rinse, and shake by tapping the strainer against the side of the sink. Then replace the seeds in the jar.

You may prefer to run the water directly into the jar. Repeat this procedure for a few day until the sprouts are ready.

There are vaieties of sprouting jars and devices on the market, some of them quite sophisticated in their capacity to maintain humidity. I recommend that you look these over at the natural food and department stores. It is also a good idea to browse through or purchase one or two of the inexpensive sprouting guides. Take your sprouting seriously. Sprouts are an important nutrient-dense food source.

Seeds can be harvested at any stage of sprouting, but "harvesting" at peak offers the highest nutrient value. One pound of some of the dried seeds will produce about eight pounds of sprouted seed. Don't be over-zealous. Don't sprout more than a tablespoonful or two at a time.

Alfalfa sprouts enhance devilled eggs.
Wheat berry sprouts add zest to fruit, crunchiness and sweetness to salads.
Soybeans simmered with fish are superb.
Lentils in soup taste like freshly ground pepper.
Garbanzos replace celery in salads.
Mung beans have the crispness of green peppers.
Mixed sprouts in vegetables add a new dimension.

Appendix D

Explaining pH

For the more technically inclined, here is a detailed explanation of pH:

In chemical parlance, pH stands for "potential" or "power" of a solution to produce positively charged hydrogen ions.

The pH number is a negative exponent. That is, pH = 7 means the concentration of positively charged hydrogen ions (H+) is 10-7 or one in ten million. This is typical of pure water. pH = 2 means that the hydrogen ion concentration is 10-2 or one in 100, characteristic of a strong acid. ph = 12 is 10-12 or one in one trillion, indicating a strong alkaline solution (because low concentration of H+ implies high concentration of OH-).

You can see that pH of a higher number means that free hydrogen ions are much more scarce; a lower number means they are more plentiful. The variation is a factor of ten for each unit change of pH.

Here's even more detail, for the few of you who are still with me:

The scale of 1 - 14 was not chosen arbitrarily. A very small percentage of water molecules ($H2O$) will naturally come apart into positively charged hydrogen ions (H+) and negatively charged hydroxyl ions (OH-). It turns out that this "dissociation constant" for water is almost exactly 10^{-14}. This means that if you multiply the concentration of H+ times the concentration of OH-, you will always get a product very close to 10^{-14}. Remember that to multiply unit numbers in exponential notation, simply add the exponents. So the exponent of the H+ concentration plus the exponent of the OH- concentration always add up to -14.

That makes the 1-14 scale very convenient: when pH is 7 (meaning the concentration of H+ is one in 10^7), then the concentration of OH- must also be one in 10^7 and the solution is chemically neutral. If the concentration of H+ is one in 10^2 (pH = 2) then the concentration of OH- must be one in 10^{12} because the two exponents have to add up to 14. Lots of extra positive ions (in this case 10^{10} times as many as negative ions) is characteristic of an acid. Similarly, a high pH means fewer H+ ions and many more OH- ions, or an alkaline solution.

Don't worry, none of this will be on a midterm. (A good tutorial on acids and pH can be found on the web at http://www.chemtutor.com/acid.htm#phbox)

Appendix E

Testimonials

Claude Larson, Chicago

"I started taking Buffered C about 2 months ago, and once I had determined the amount that my body likes, which is 4 to 5 1/2 teaspoons spaced throughout the day, the true effects became evident. Good, consistent, calm energy, with the added side effect of reducing cravings. I highly recommend Buffered C."

~~~~

Pearl Harris, New York

"I lost eleven pounds, and wondered why. I did nothing to change my diet. Then I remembered I had been taking that buffered C/mineral formula."

~~~~

Elise Zurlo, Clinical Nutritionist, Florida

"At one point, I had been suffering from extreme food-allergy-related anxiety after every meal. Buffered Vitamin C Powder was the only thing that gave me relief. I have to take it before meals to stop the reaction before it starts. I also use Buffered Vitamin C to stop other allergic reactions. Typically, any allergic reaction I am suffering from will pass within 10 minutes of taking the Buffered Vitamin C. If the reaction is severe and doesn't pass on the first dose, I will take additional doses every 20 minutes until the reaction has passed. Another helpful hint is that it works even better if mixed with chilled water, although it works for me with room temperature water.

I always travel with Buffered Vitamin C and I always keep several extra bottles on hand so that I never run out. It is truly one of my most important supplements.

Buffered Vitamin C is truly the most effective allergy relief I have ever had . . . and I've been allergic since the day I was born."

~~~~~

Patient S.J., Novato, California

"This happened to me 28 years ago, and I remember it like yesterday. In 1975, I was admitted to the ecological unit of Henrotin Hospital in Chicago, because I was extremely suicidal and was suffering from clinical depression.

"My attending physician was Dr. Theron Randolph, who was the pioneering head of the ecological unit. To diagnose the source of my mental state, Dr. Randolph started by testing me for food allergies. I was tested for one food at a time. When I was given wheat to eat, within 20 minutes my pulse accelerated 100 beats. I began convulsing and threatened to jump out the window right then and there. It took four nurses to restrain me. Shortly after the nurses restrained me, Dr. Randolph came in and intervened by giving me an infusion of a mixture he called 'salts.'

"Within an hour of receiving this infusion, my system was back to normal and I felt a lot better. It was quite a remarkable experience. The 'salts' neutralized my severe reaction to wheat and brought me back to normal.The next day one of the nurses told me that just as I was having my wheat reaction, one of Dr. Randolph's largest financial donors was admitted to the hospital suffering from a heart attack. Dr. Randolph assured himself that the man was being given proper care by his colleagues, and he came running up to the unit to help me. According to the nurse, he elected to stay with me through my horrible ordeal.

"I thought this was a very kind and professional deed. I believe his kindness and his "salts" contributed greatly to my recovery."

[This case history comes from a patient and demonstrates that the alkali salts could reverse an acute reaction to wheat, that caused pyschiatric, "suicidal' tendencies. since the development of buffered C, it has replaced the salts.]

~~~~~

Gabriel Cousins, MD, New Mexico

"I have been using buffered vitamin C for addiction for years. It really works to control symptoms for my patients."

~~~~~

Vivian Smith, Salt Lake City, Utah

"When I get a wild allergic sneezing spell, I immediately take some of the calcium/buffered C product in a little water and hold it under my tongue for faster absorption. It works like a charm, every time."

~~~~~

Debbie Halpern, Dallas, Texas

"It was the only product that helped me stop smoking."

pH Testing
Information

After following the instructions on the next page, the testing paper will turn a certain color. This can be matched against the color chart in the envelope. The color of the paper indicates acidity or alkalinity, as measured on a scale of 5.5 to 8.0.

Using saliva as the testing medium, a healthy pH is about 6.8 to 7.2. The yellow range on the pH paper indicates an acidic pH below 6.5. This test roughly indicates the pH of internal body fluids.

Keep in mind that the test may not always be accurate. Saliva could be influenced by food you have eaten (which is the reason testing should be done first thing in the morning). However, if you repeat the test several times, you will have a gauge that could be fairly accurate.

An interesting experiment would be to check your results *before* you start using the *California Calcium Countdown* formula, or something similar, and then check your pH again a couple of weeks later. You may be very pleasantly surprised.

Never use the testing papers internally.

pH Testing
Instructions

Saliva pH can be affected by food and drink, so the pH test should be performed after at least two hours of strict fasting. (You should be eating frequently and drinking water even more frequently, so the best time for the test is first thing in the morning, before anything has gone into your rmouth.) pH should be tested over a period of several days to make sure you have a consistent reading. Follow these steps to measure saliva pH:

1) Swallow a few times to induce your salivary glands to make a fresh mouthful.

2) Spit a small sample of saliva onto a plate.

3) Dunk one end of a pH test strip into the saliva to saturate it (do not put the test strip in your mouth - it is only approved for use outside the body).

4) Shake off the excess liquid.

5) Within 30 seconds after the strip first gets wet, find the box on the color chart that is the closest color match. The number above the box is your saliva pH.

Please see test-
ing information
on previous two
pages.

Never use the
testing strips
internally.